Back to Life
After a Heart Crisis

❖

Back to Life
After a Heart Crisis

A Doctor and His Wife
Share Their 8-Step Cardiac Comeback Plan

MARC WALLACK, M.D., AND JAMIE COLBY
with
ALISA BOWMAN

AVERY
a member of
Penguin Group (USA) Inc.
New York

Published by the Penguin Group
Penguin Group (USA) Inc., 375 Hudson Street, New York, New York 10014, USA ·
Penguin Group (Canada), 90 Eglinton Avenue East, Suite 700, Toronto, Ontario M4P 2Y3, Canada
(a division of Pearson Penguin Canada Inc.) · Penguin Books Ltd, 80 Strand, London WC2R 0RL, England ·
Penguin Ireland, 25 St Stephen's Green, Dublin 2, Ireland (a division of Penguin Books Ltd) ·
Penguin Group (Australia), 250 Camberwell Road, Camberwell, Victoria 3124, Australia
(a division of Pearson Australia Group Pty Ltd) · Penguin Books India Pvt Ltd,
11 Community Centre, Panchsheel Park, New Delhi–110 017, India ·
Penguin Group (NZ), 67 Apollo Drive, Rosedale, North Shore 0632, New Zealand
(a division of Pearson New Zealand Ltd) · Penguin Books (South Africa) (Pty) Ltd,
24 Sturdee Avenue, Rosebank, Johannesburg 2196, South Africa

Penguin Books Ltd, Registered Offices: 80 Strand, London WC2R 0RL, England

Most Avery books are available at special quantity discounts for bulk
purchase for sales promotions, premiums, fund-raising, and educational needs.
Special books or book excerpts also can be created to fit specific needs. For details, write
Penguin Group (USA) Inc. Special Markets, 375 Hudson Street, New York, NY 10014.

Library of Congress Cataloging-in-Publication Data

Wallack, Marc K.
Back to life after a heart crisis : a doctor and his wife share their 8-step cardiac comeback plan /
Marc Wallack and Jamie Colby with Alisa Bowman.
p.   cm.
Includes bibliographical references and index.
ISBN 978-1-58333-367-9
1. Heart—Diseases—Popular works.   2. Heart—Diseases—Psychological aspects.
3. Wallack, Marc K.—Health.   4. Physicians—Diseases—New York—Psychological aspects.
I. Colby, Jamie.   II. Bowman, Alisa.   III. Title.
RC672.W35   2010   2009040972
616.1'2—dc22

Printed in the United States of America
1   3   5   7   9   10   8   6   4   2

BOOK DESIGN BY TANYA MAIBORODA

*Penguin is committed to publishing works of quality and integrity.
In that spirit, we are proud to offer this book to our readers;
however, the story, the experiences, and the words
are the authors' alone.*

From Marc to Jamie and Jamie to Marc:
It takes two to make a comeback.

Contents

Acknowledgments

WE FRANKLY NEVER EXPECTED TO WRITE THIS BOOK, BUT WHEN WE could not find anything on the shelf to help us through a cardiac recovery— especially one that covered the emotional, physical, and professional toll it took on both of us—we knew we had to. Still, we would not have been able to share with you what we learned without the help and support of the caring people whom we must introduce you to here.

Cardiac surgeon Sam Lang was someone Marc, as the Chairman of Surgery, had recruited. Beyond his superb technical skill, we quickly learned that Sam was also a kind and compassionate man. Our thanks to you, Sam, for saving Marc's life and performing the quadruple bypass that allowed Marc to run more marathons and truly enjoy the rest of his life. Many thanks go to Sari and Dr. Arthur Agatston for Arthur's early care of Marc in

Miami and for their support of our book. Dr. Isadore Rosenfeld has been as supportive as a family member.

Alisa Bowman heard our voice and helped us write in it. With multiple *New York Times* bestsellers under her belt, she showed great passion for our story and believed in our desire to help others struggling to build their own cardiac comeback.

We'll never forget publisher Megan Newman's and senior editor Lucia Watson's response during our first visit to publisher Avery/Penguin. "You had us at hello!" they exclaimed at the end of the hour in which we'd laughed, cried, and somehow felt at ease enough to detail our first sexual experience after surgery. Megan and Lucia believed in our desire to give all heart disease patients the tools to reclaim their life completely. Lucia's guidance enhanced our comeback plan to guarantee that a heart disease survivor's next chapter in life will be even better than the first.

Bill Shinker, Lisa Johnson, Miriam Rich, and Lindsay Gordon all played key roles in bringing this book to life. Our sincere thanks for their encouragement, expertise, and genuine enthusiasm for our story.

Through our experience and Marc's recovery, we quickly learned that it takes two to make a cardiac comeback. Our blessing was finding each other twenty years ago and sharing our life together. We're convinced we would not have survived Marc's cardiac recovery without each other's shoulders to lean on. If we inspire you to do just one thing in your own recovery (though in this book we know you'll find much more), identify one special person who will be there to hold you when you need to cry, ask health professionals the questions you may not think to ask, and tell those who are insensitive to walk the other way. It's just one of our life preservers that you'll find in *Back to Life*.

Our children, our parents, and especially each of our brothers, Jonathan Colby and the late Alan Davis, refused to let us give up both physically and emotionally when on so many occasions that seemed the only option. We will never forget your inspiration, love, and support. We cherish our friends who understood so often that there were good days and bad, easy ones and ones too difficult to handle. We can't name all of you here but note with special gratitude Dr. Harvey Yavil, Rena Shectman, and Rabbi Richard Address. Thanks for being there every time we needed you.

Marc's special thanks go to his team of Margie Anderson, Olga Rosado, Dr. John Degliuomini, and Dr. Will Wang. Throughout Marc's recovery, they reminded him he was still the leader he'd been before his heart disease diagnosis, only healthier. The New York Medical College students and the St. Vincent's Manhattan surgical residents whom Marc recruited still bring strength and smiles to his mended heart.

Marc's former patient Robert Facchina gave us both something unique. On a day Marc was so down he was unable to get up from the couch, Bob, a melanoma cancer survivor due to Marc's first melanoma vaccine, detailed how he'd lived his own "Chapter 2," turning our doom and gloom into determination to live a better, stronger, and more rewarding life even after a heart disease diagnosis. Bob, the mosaic you gave us is a wonderful reminder of that extraordinary day.

Taking time off to help in Marc's cardiac comeback was no easy task for Jamie, who works in a business where showing up every day counts. During those sometimes unimaginable days at home, work was her best medicine. Immense thanks to Jamie's special mentors and friends, including FOX News Channel CEO Roger Ailes and FOX attorney Dianne Brandi. You were among the first to understand the importance of our writing this book and sharing our experience. Your support and kindness all these years mean so much to us. Our sincerest thanks go also to Bill Shine,

Suzanne Scott, Michael Clemente, Peter Johnson, Jr., David Clark, and others in Jamie's FOX family.

And finally, we realize our experience may have been extreme, but we really must thank the people who weren't as kind or understanding as we would have liked. As it turns out, without your missteps we would have never learned the survival skills we offer other heart disease patients in *Back to Life* so they can achieve their own cardiac comeback . . . our proven path to physical, emotional, and professional wellness . . . in just eight steps.

To your health,

Marc Wallack, M.D., and Jamie Colby

❖ PART ONE ❖

The Hope

Introduction

You: Back and Better Than Ever

IT DOESN'T MATTER WHY YOU ARE HOLDING THIS BOOK. IT DOESN'T matter if you ended up here because your cholesterol topped 300 or your blood pressure hit 220/120. It doesn't matter if, like me, you ignored that chest pain for minutes, hours, or even days, telling yourself that it wasn't angina or a heart attack, but rather indigestion or food poisoning. It doesn't matter how many bypass grafts you now have or will soon have on your arteries. It doesn't matter how much your heart muscle has been damaged.

No matter what medicines you are taking or artificial hardware you may have installed inside your body, there's hope. There's help. There's the rest of your life waiting to be lived.

Back to Life After a Heart Crisis can help, no matter what kind of major cardiac problem you've experienced, from severe angina to heart bypass surgery to heart vessel stenting to transplant to angioplasty to heart attack. It can help you no matter how out of shape you are or how unhealthy your current lifestyle is. It can help no matter how incapacitated you feel.

Back to Life After a Heart Crisis can help you no matter what. All you need is this: hope for something better. That's it. As both a doctor and a patient, I'll give you the tools you need to turn that hope into the rest of your life.

You have another chance.

You can make a comeback.

You can live a fulfilling life again.

You can feel productive, strong, loved, understood, respected, and worthwhile again. You can overcome the anxiety, the anger, the sadness, the guilt, and the regret. And, yes, you can even get past that paralyzing fear of death.

I know you can because I did. I've been exactly where you are right now. I've been in that hospital bed. I've worn that paper gown. I've had my chest bone cracked open, my heart stopped, and my breathing controlled by a machine.

I've faced that long recovery. I've had to find a way to get to sleep at night. Yes, I know about that horrible fear, of not knowing whether or not you will wake up after closing your eyes or of not knowing whether or not the big one will hit while you are having sex with your wife.

I know about the frustration that surfaces when people treat you like damaged goods or ask over and over again in a tone that can't help but sound condescending, "How are you feeling?"

I know about that sensation of letting everyone down.

I know about the self-loathing, of wondering, "Why would anyone want to stay married to someone like me?"

I know it. I've lived it. I've been there.

Two and a half years after undergoing quadruple bypass surgery, I did something that stunned my coworkers and friends. I ran a marathon. Only about 1 percent of the population ever runs a marathon. Even fewer do so after being diagnosed with heart disease. I'm not telling you that you have to run a marathon. I'm just here to tell you this: Anything is possible after heart disease. Anything.

Here's what else I know: There is more to your life than this hospital bed, this bypass graft, this valve, this stent, or this medication. You have not reached the end of your book of life. You have what it takes to live another chapter, and another, and another. You are strong enough, good enough, and resilient enough.

You are. You really are.

Your life is not over. Rather, it has just begun.

A Little About Me

I am a surgical oncologist, a Vice Chairman and Professor of Surgery at New York Medical College, and Chief of the Department of Surgery at Metropolitan Hospital in New York City.

I'm a cancer expert. I developed and led one of the first highly publicized cancer vaccine trials to treat melanoma, the deadliest type of skin cancer in the world. Right now I am working on launching a second trial of a new, more powerful vaccine I developed for melanoma.

I know that serious illness changes people because I've seen it happen to patient after patient during the more than thirty years of my professional career. I have always believed that I am responsible not only for what goes on inside a patient's body in the operating room, but also for what goes on inside a patient's head after leaving the hospital. Since my first days as a surgeon, I've visited my patients after surgery, to check on not only their physical recovery, but their emotional recovery as well. I ask them about their pain, their fears, their doubts, and their anger. I tirelessly work to help them live again *emotionally* after I've done the necessary surgery to help them live *physically*. Throughout the medical community, I'm known for my careful follow-up of my surgical patients.

Despite all of this, I was not prepared for how serious illness would change *me*. I was a doctor. I knew how to help patients. I didn't know how to be one. I never expected that I would need my own doctor, my own therapist, and my own team of confidants so I could recover emotionally from surgery.

I didn't learn about being a patient in medical school. I didn't learn about it during my residency. I didn't learn about it during my many years of medical practice. I learned it by living it.

Being a heart disease patient taught me a lot.

Being a patient taught me about denial. I'm not a cardiologist, but you would think that all my years of medical training would have ensured that I knew the difference between angina (chest pain) and indigestion. They didn't. When I felt chest pain during a run one evening about a week before my bypass, I tried to push through it. Then I eventually walked back to my apartment and took Tums. When the same thing happened during a run the next day, I took Maalox. When it happened the next day, too, I took Nexium, Tums, and Maalox. The following day? I added Prevacid to the mix. *I thought I was too important, too invincible, and too necessary to have heart disease.* I didn't have time for heart disease. I had so many sick patients to care for and so many surgical residents and medical students to teach!

Being a heart disease patient taught me about vulnerability. I learned what it felt like to be poked and prodded. I experienced the embarrassment of having my own staff—people I supervised and trained—care for me while I was incapacitated. One of my resident physicians had to give me a rectal exam before my surgery. Let me tell you: The experience wasn't a walk in the park for either one of us.

It taught me about fear. I remember just how scared I was at St. Vincent's Hospital Manhattan just before my surgery. I remember how scared I was so, so many times afterward, too.

It taught me about guilt, anxiety, anger, and sadness, too.

I must have experienced every single negative emotion there was to experience. Every. Single. One. I learned about all of them.

But I didn't give up. My life got better. Now I'm stronger, happier, and healthier than ever.

I've learned from this experience. Now I want to teach you everything that I learned so you can emerge stronger, happier, and healthier, too.

What You'll Get out of This Book

Back to Life After a Heart Crisis offers inspiration coupled with a step-by-step program for creating a new and improved life. I like to think of it as Lance Armstrong's *It's Not About the Bike* meets *Heart Disease for Dummies* meets *The Doctors Book of Home Remedies*. Throughout the pages of this book, you'll find a step-by-step map that will take you from point A—where you are right now—to point B—the new, improved, and courageous you. You will find:

- **An eight-step plan for conquering your fear of living.** After a major cardiac event, it's normal for everyday experiences such as walking down a crowded street, showing up for a doctor's appointment, or driving a car to lead to panic. It's normal for any activity that increases heart rate—from climbing a flight of stairs to a treadmill stress test—to trigger anxiety. You don't have to live with these fears, though. You can overcome them. You can get back to living. To do so, you'll face each and every one of these anxiety-producing situations. In Part 2 of this book, you'll find a series of chapters devoted to the most common fears of heart disease survivors. To make a full recovery and live life to the fullest, I recommend that you face these fears one step at a time. I'll be right there with you every step of the way, teaching you the fundamentals that helped me.

- **Answers to all the questions you are too afraid or embarrassed to ask.** Do you want to know how to overcome your fear of death so you can rekindle your sex life? Do you want to know ways to get back to sleep at night? How about overcoming the anxiety of doctors' visits and test results? And what do you say to all of those well-meaning people who make comments and ask questions that put you on the defensive? You'll find answers to those questions, and many more.

- **Inspirational stories from me and other heart disease survivors.** I'll tell you about a guy who was once hooked up to an artificial heart machine and now runs triathlons. And a type-A woman who was so career driven that she asked her husband to bring her laptop to the hospital, where she'd been admitted for chest pain. I'll explain how she learned to reduce her work stress. And there's the story of the man with a heart rhythm abnormality that has caused him to have multiple near-death experiences. That's right. He's seen the tunnel, heard the harps, and come back to tell us all about it. Is death as scary as we all think? Read his story to find out.

- **Help for the people who love you most.** It's not easy taking care of us heart disease survivors. About 75 percent of caregivers report feeling strained emotionally, physically, and financially. Compared to non-caregivers, they have a higher amount of stress hormones circulating in their bloodstreams and, as a result, have weakened immunity and a higher risk of experiencing anxiety and/or depression. They may eventually develop long-term medical problems, such as heart disease and cancer. My wife, FOX News Channel Anchor and attorney Jamie Colby, cared for me during my recovery. Throughout the pages of this book, she offers her advice to help caregivers survive this experience with you—without suffering undue stress in the process. For instance, one of her first caregiver tips in Chapter 2 will help you figure out what to do when you learn that your loved one has heart disease.

- **The specific advice you need to get better and stay better.** You'll find delicious and easy-to-make heart-healthy recipes, an extensive heart-healthy restaurant eating guide (one you *can* follow), exercise plans, destressing advice, and more. It's everything you need to go from the doctor's office to the rest of your life!

- **A unique challenge.** I will challenge you to do something truly amazing, something that proves to you, and others around you, that you are back and better than ever. I'll challenge you to take on a major physical accomplishment such as a walkathon, endurance cycling event, mountain climb, long-distance bike ride, hike on the Appalachian Trail, or another symbolic feat. You may wonder why the eight-step plan must culminate with a physical challenge. Isn't it enough to just be alive? Isn't it enough to have survived a major cardiac event? For many survivors, the answer is no. Most of us need proof that we really are alive. Most of us, after we claw our way back to good health and after our physicians tell us that every part of our bodies is in perfect working order, still have doubts. Physical accomplishments help you say yes. Yes, I'm back. Yes, I'm alive. Yes, I really can enjoy life again.

You can find the courage to face the everyday tasks that make life worth living. I'll show you how. I'll help you to become a stronger person, one who loves life and who is no longer afraid. I'll help you get to that next chapter in the book of your life. This isn't your end. It's just your beginning. Have the courage to turn the page.

❖ CHAPTER ❖

1

The Story of This Courageous Survivor

THE VAST MAJORITY OF US ARE QUITE CONTENT TO LIVE OUR LIVES in denial—tricking ourselves into believing that life as we know it will go on forever. When a doctor mentions the words "blocked coronary arteries," it can feel as if we just got punched in the stomach. We'd rather not have to come to terms with what is really going on in our bodies.

I began to feel, and tried to ignore, an eerie sensation that something was wrong a few days before my diagnosis. During one run after work, I felt pain in my chest, roughly seven minutes into the run. I brushed it off as gastric reflux and stress. "I had a really stressful day at work," I told myself. I walked home and it went away.

The next day it happened again. "It's really severe reflux. Maybe I have an ulcer," I told myself.

When I noticed the pain, yet again, on the third run, I decided I must be getting it because I was trying to run indoors on a treadmill! I thought, "If I just push through this, it will go away."

But it would only go away once I stopped running. That was a sign. It should have tipped me off. I should have known better.

Then, on the fourth day, I was running in Central Park. Roughly seven minutes into the run I felt a pain in my chest that radiated to my chin and down my left arm. I'm a doctor. I knew about chest pain that radiates to the left arm. It usually means one thing, and that one thing has nothing to do with heartburn.

I knew that, but I didn't want to know it. So I tried to convince myself that it was nothing, that it was really acid reflux.

A little voice whispered, "Marc, this is not normal." I answered that voice by walking home and taking an antacid. I soon felt better, so much better that, when I saw my wife getting ready to go out for a bike ride, I said, "Can I go with you?"

She looked at me as if I was crazy and said, "Relax. It's your day off. Go lie down."

The little voice whispered again, "Something is wrong. This isn't right."

I answered it, "Okay, okay, this is probably nothing, but I'll call my cardiologist, okay?"

I made an appointment with him for the next morning. Then I went out to dinner to celebrate my mother's eighty-eighth birthday.

The next morning, I went to the operating room to remove an apple-size mass on the left thigh of one of my patients. The one-hour procedure went well. As I operated, I continually made a mental note of how my chest felt. Operating is stressful. If I'd really had something wrong with my heart, I would have felt pain during the operation. I didn't. My chest didn't hurt at all. I felt alert. I felt normal. I felt like my old self.

"See?" I told that voice, "I'm fine. This is nothing. I'm fine."

Afterward, in my suit and tie, I decided to walk to my cardiologist's appointment. The hospital was on Twelfth Street and Seventh Avenue. My doctor's office was on Twenty-third Street and Sixth Avenue. That's twelve blocks, or about one half a mile. It was 93 degrees.

Six minutes into the walk, I started to sweat and feel that sensation in my chest again.

I stopped into a convenience store and bought some Maalox and a large bottle of cold water. The pain subsided again, but I was finally concerned.

A short time later, my cardiologist put me on a treadmill for a stress test. Three minutes into the test, my doctor stopped the treadmill. I still had nine minutes left. A typical stress test lasts twelve minutes. Something was wrong. I knew it before he told me.

The EKG showed a pattern that indicated that my heart was not getting enough oxygen. It meant that I was not the healthy marathoner I'd thought I was. It meant that my life would not go on forever. It meant that I was not invincible.

It was more information than I ever wanted to know about the state of affairs inside my body.

My doctor recommended that I undergo an immediate angiogram. He told me that I needed to get to the hospital, and that I should call someone to drive me. When I called Jamie, at the time a CBS television reporter and anchor, she was just getting off the air.

The rest is a jumble of random memories and thoughts. Thank God Jamie was there to ask the important questions and hear and remember the answers, because my mind was elsewhere. It was racing, "This can't be happening. I'm healthy. Just yesterday I was running. No, this is a mistake. It can't be happening. Me? Blocked arteries? It's a mistake." It was like an out-of-body experience. I just kept thinking, "This cannot be happening to me."

Except it wasn't a mistake, and it was happening to me.

Later that same day, a physician—a colleague I worked with and who cleared some of my patients for surgery—inserted a catheter into my leg and guided it to the blood vessels near my heart. The room at my hospital was filled to capacity with concerned coworkers. They crowded in front of a monitor that displayed real-time photos of the insides of my coronary arteries. When I heard a nun say, "Oh, Jesus," Jamie and I knew things were serious.

All of my coronary arteries were more than 95 percent blocked. I needed a surgeon to harvest healthy blood vessels from my leg and one from my chest, sewing them to the diseased ones leading to my heart. I needed a quadruple bypass, and I needed it quickly.

The Doctor Becomes a Patient

Two days later, I was on a gurney outside the operating room. I realized that I'd never before looked at the hospital ceiling. What I saw wasn't pretty.

"Gee, these lights are ugly," I thought as they wheeled me to the operating room. I'd stood in this room just days before, only I wasn't the patient. I was the surgeon. The cardiac team had not needed the room, so I'd used it to do a modified radical mastectomy for a woman with advanced breast cancer.

Now I wasn't the person wearing the blue gown and mask and holding a scalpel. I was the guy who would soon be unconscious and nearly naked on the table. I was the guy who would have the iodine preparation on his chest and legs. I would be stained a deep burnt orange. I'd have a breathing tube down my throat.

My chief of cardiac surgery, someone I'd recruited to work at the hospital a few years before, was going to crack open my breastbone, spread apart my ribs, and take my aorta (the main artery that carries blood from the heart to smaller arteries throughout the body) and another large vein and attach both to a machine that would pump oxygenated blood throughout my body. This machine would temporarily function as my heart.

He was going to stop my heart.

Then he was going to take a vein from my leg and divide it into three veins and use them and a major artery running down the center of chest bone to bypass the four blockages in my coronary arteries that supply blood to make my heart muscle pump.

It was serious stuff.

I knew about the risks of this surgery. I knew that any number of techniques used during the surgery could cause a clot to dislodge and travel into a smaller artery, triggering a stroke in my brain or a life-threatening blockage in my lungs. I knew that I could suffer a heart attack soon after the procedure. I also knew that some hearts refused to be shocked back to life.

I knew about so many possible problems. I'd heard them recounted many times every week when I presided over the hospital's Morbidity and Mortality Conference. During these meetings surgeons and staff dissect what went wrong during various hospital procedures that resulted in complications or, in the worst-case scenario, death. I knew that surgical battles didn't always end in typical Hollywood style. I knew that sometimes the good guys lost, that sometimes good patients—patients who should have lived—died, because of some random chance.

As the anesthesia clouded my thinking and made my eyelids heavy, I hoped and prayed that I would not be one of those patients. I hoped and prayed that I would be able to open my eyes once more.

I'm Alive, but Who Am I Really?

Four bypassed arteries and twelve hours later, I woke from the haze of anesthesia. I was in the intensive care unit. Wires held my breastbone together. Fine thread held my new grafts to my coronary arteries.

I took a breath. "That's good," I thought. My breathing tube was out.

I'd instructed my medical team to keep me under anesthesia until they could remove my breathing tube. If I'd woken with a tube still in my throat, I would have known instantly that something had gone wrong.

Thank God for that air. Thank God for my eyes. They were open. I was alive. I'd made it. There were wires and tubes sticking out of my chest. A temporary pacemaker was attached to my heart. I was in a drug-induced fog. I felt nothing.

I saw my wife, Jamie. Our eyes met, and, without words, we read each other's thoughts: "*We still have more time together.*"

For that I was happy.

A New Man

It wasn't until twenty-four hours later, when I left the ICU for a regular hospital room, that I realized I would need more than wires and thread to hold myself together. I would need a special kind of resilience, too. That realization came when I saw my children. They looked at me with loving expressions, but I could see fear in their eyes.

It was then that I realized that the first part of my life had ended . . . forever.

Every single aspect of who I was as a man, surgeon, husband, father, and runner had shifted while I'd been on that table. It had all changed, in just a few hours. In just twelve hours, a chapter of my life had come to an end. In just twelve hours, my life had drastically changed. In just twelve hours, I'd become a completely different person, and that person was a stranger to me.

When I'd been wheeled into the operating room, I'd been a doctor. I'd been Marc Wallack, M.D., a top-of-my-field surgeon, administrator, and researcher.

When I'd been wheeled into that room, I'd been Marc Wallack, the strong family man who listened to, comforted, and solved the world's problems for my wife, my kids, and my mother.

When I'd been wheeled into that room, I'd been Marc Wallack, the incredibly fit and healthy marathoner.

I'd been in control.

Now the only part of the old me that remained was my name. I hadn't died, but I might as well have. I was a new person, whether I wanted to embrace that person or not.

One day I was running in Central Park, training for my next marathon, noticing chest pain and a tingling sensation in my chin that I told myself was gastric reflux. On another I was recovering from surgery. One day I was strong. Then next I was weak. One day I could run a marathon. The next I couldn't get out of bed without assistance. One day my colleagues looked up to me. The next they seemed to see me as weak and "damaged."

One day I was the family rock. The next I was the family's project.

One day I took life for granted. The next I found myself hoping and praying that there would be more to my life than just one chapter, that I not only would survive this, but also have something to survive for.

If I'm Still Alive, Why Do I Feel Dead?

My cardiologist assured me that I would recover most if not all of my physical abilities. Part of me believed this. Another part of me didn't. I was afraid. *Will I be able to get well enough to go home? When I get home, will I be able to function independently? Will I be able to become a successful member of the medical community again or is my career over? What will happen to me if I can't go back to work? Will I be able to pay the mortgage on my home? Will I ever have an appetite again? Will I ever want to have sex again? Will I be able to run again? Will I be able to be a good husband or father again? Will my wife become overwhelmed and fed up with taking care of me and leave me for a healthier man? If that happens, will I be able to go on living?*

During each of the four nights of my hospital stay, I would hear my heart beating. *Keep beating. Keep beating. Please keep beating.* After finally falling asleep, I would wake from a night terror, drenched in sweat with my heart racing to 120 or 130 beats per minute, even though my resting pulse should have been between 80 and 90.

❀   JAMIE'S ADVICE FOR CAREGIVERS   ❀

So many people send flowers to hospital patients, but flowers can be more depressing than uplifting. Marc, for instance, said that the flowers made him feel sicker. He didn't want to see himself as the type of person who needed other people's sympathy. So we put Marc's flowers in the hallway and we had so many that they lined both sides, from his room to the nurses' station.

Instead I decorated his room with comforting objects from home. I brought in a miniature waterfall and CD player to drown out the beeping and other hospital sounds. I brought in some photos, too. I tried to make his room seem as much like home as possible.

During the first six weeks after surgery, I became depressed and withdrawn. I had no appetite. I lost fifteen pounds in just two weeks, and more in the weeks that followed. I did not want to talk to friends who called to see how I was doing. I became annoyed by well-meaning comments about how I looked or questions about how I was feeling.

The slightest reminders of the angina that led to my surgery sent me into a panic. I was *terrified* of doing anything—even walking quickly or uphill or exerting myself in any way—that would speed my heart rate.

I did not want to leave the apartment. I did not want to exercise. I did not want to eat. I began using my pain medication to medicate myself emotionally—to take away the mental pain I felt about my illness.

I was an emotional wreck.

Choose to Live

It took some time, but eventually I was able to take the part of me that had changed for the *worse* and create a new me who had changed for the *better*. The first part of my life had come to an end. It was time to define and build the new Marc. If I wanted to embrace the next stage, I had to get started.

This metamorphosis started about two weeks after my surgery, when I read Lance Armstrong's *It's Not About the Bike*. It gave me courage. I knew that when I was ready to engage in life again, I was not going to be a victim. I made a decision. I decided to live—to face my many fears and create a new and better life. I decided to write and then live the next chapter of my life. During the next two and a half years, that's what I did. I rebuilt my health. I rebuilt my family relationships. I rebuilt my career. I rebuilt my identity. I did it by facing and overcoming each of my fears, starting with the fears that were easiest to handle and most important to my daily survival and working my way up to the ones that seemed hardest to face.

I emerged a better, stronger, healthier, happier person.

Looking back on the Marc Wallack of 2002, it's amazing to me that I found the will to go on. I think about that man, the one who felt so weak, alone, and misunderstood. He was sick. He was underweight. He was terrified of living.

Then I contrast that image with the Marc Wallack of today. I see a happier man who appreciates life more. I see a whole person, someone who balances work and life. I'm a better physician than I was. I better understand my patients. I'm a better husband. I'm a better father.

Heart disease has taught me something important. It has taught me how to live my life with courage, integrity, and meaning and, if I accomplish nothing else with this book, I can teach you to reclaim your life, too.

You can transform yourself from a survivor living in fear to a courageous survivor who loves life. You can move beyond fearing the future (*when will the big one hit?*) to creating your future. You can do more than hope for a second chapter of your life. You can live it.

2

An Insider's Guide to Early Cardiac Care

I'M ABOUT TO TAKE YOU ON A TRIP, ONE THAT STARTS AT THE moment of diagnosis and does not end until many days, months, or years afterward. Just how long the trip will last depends on a number of factors— the severity of your heart disease, your state of mind, the quality of your relationships, and, most important, just how badly you want to reclaim your life.

It doesn't matter precisely where you are on that journey—whether you just got word that you need a stent or a bypass, whether you are about to be discharged after having a heart attack, or whether your physical recovery took place more than a year ago. No matter where you draw your starting line, your journey will span the same basic route.

In this chapter, I start the journey at the beginning, offering you advice that can help you the moment you learn of your diagnosis. You'll find advice for how to pick a hospital, how to make the best of your hospital recovery time, and even how to get from the hospital to your home in the least stressful way possible. You'll find everything you need here for those first steps toward your starting line.

Then, in Part 2 of this book, I'll fire the starter's pistol, and you'll start moving toward the finish line, one step at a time.

◈ JAMIE'S ADVICE FOR CAREGIVERS ◈

After Marc and I learned that his coronaries were 95 percent blocked, I turned to him and asked, "What should we do?" I did not feel equipped to make a decision. I was scared. Did he need surgery right away? Was a bypass better than a stent or an angioplasty? Should we do whatever his cardiologist recommended?

You will probably feel just as scared when you first hear the diagnosis of heart disease. Know that, as I learned, you do not—in the vast majority of cases—have to make a decision right away. Unless your loved one's life is in imminent danger, you have time. Weigh your options. Gather information. Seek out second, third, and fourth opinions.

How to Pick a Hospital and Surgeon

Some of you reading this book may be just discovering that you have heart disease and you need to make some choices. This section is for you. Perhaps your doctor recommends surgery, but you wonder whether you can manage your condition with medication. Perhaps your doctor recommends a stent, but you wonder if you should just bite the bullet and get the bypass.

Here's what to do, and it's the kind of advice that only a doctor who has lived through this can give you. Before agreeing on any procedure, get three opinions. If they do not concur, choose bypass surgery over an angioplasty or stent. Bypass surgery may be more invasive and have a longer recovery time, but it tends to result in longer-lasting good health. Many patients who undergo angioplasty or stenting need a follow-up procedure within two to four years. Believe me, you want this to be your last trip to the hospital. You want to walk away from this experience knowing you are fixed. You don't want to be continually wondering, "When will this stop working?"

The only procedure that can provide that kind of peace of mind is a bypass. That's why I chose one.

I had other choices, of course. One cardiologist told me, "If it were me, I would not opt for surgery. I would get multiple stents." When he said that, I looked at him incredulously and said, "But I have a lot of blockages. It's pretty extensive."

He told me that the stents were all I needed. I told him I'd think about it and I got another opinion. This time I asked a cardiac surgeon. He bluntly said, "Marc, it's time to go to the OR."

I said, "But the cardiologist told me that stents were all I needed."

He was someone I knew well. He said, "Marc, do you think I would operate on you if it wasn't necessary?"

I said, "No, I don't." But I got a third opinion anyway, this time from a well-known cardiac surgeon with one of the most prestigious hospitals in New York. He said, "So when do we drape you and operate?"

I scheduled myself for a bypass.

Of course, it's a big operation. The good news is this: It usually saves lives rather than ends them. Fewer than 3 percent of people die on the table or soon after.

You can increase your odds of survival by picking the best surgeon and hospital for your bypass, angioplasty, or stenting. Some hospitals have much better success rates than others. The top hospitals have a bypass death rate of just 1.4 percent, whereas the worst ones have a death rate that's around 6.5 percent. This is your life we're talking about, so it makes good sense to shop around for a hospital that has a good track record, one with a death rate closer to 2 than to 6. You can find out the success and death rates for various hospitals by checking any number of institutions that offer health-care "report cards." I've listed a number of these companies in Chapter 13.

Also, make sure your hospital is accredited and houses a cardiac center. Do not make the mistake of choosing a low-volume hospital just because it's close to home. Ask how many bypasses the cardiac center does a year. The number should be at least two hundred.

Pick a surgeon who:

- Is board-certified in the field of open-heart surgery. To do so, check the lists of board-certified cardiothoracic surgeons in the American Board of Medical Specialties (ABMS) annual directory, available online at www.abms.org. Also, the letters FACS should appear after his or her name. This means that the doctor is a Fellow of the American College of Surgeons, and adds another layer of certification.
- Specializes in heart surgery. Ask how many surgeries he or she does a year. The number should be between one hundred and two hundred.
- Is recommended by others. Ask the opinion of other surgeons in your area along with other heart disease survivors.
- Has a good track record. The surgeon's mortality rate (total number of deaths) of less than 2 percent and a morbidity rate (total number of adverse complications that result in long-term poor health) between 5 and 7 percent. To find this information, use any number of health-care report card services. Also I've listed them for you in Chapter 13.

During the Days Leading Up to Surgery

If you are about to undergo a bypass, angioplasty, or another surgical procedure to fix your heart, do the following before you go to the hospital if you are able to prepare.

Line up support. Don't do this alone. No army commander goes into battle without backup. Those who go willingly go with teams of trusted associates at their side, protecting them and moving them forward toward a common goal. In my case, my team was my wife, my mother, my children, my brother, my brother-in-law, my in-laws, select friends and colleagues, certain professionals, and a higher power that helped me fight, and helped me find and claim a "Chapter 2" of my life.

You need a similar support team. You won't know the names of everyone on your support team now, but you do need to identify at least one person. It should be someone who can hold your hand from this point forward, someone who is calm enough to ask those important questions and hear those important answers, someone who is strong and assertive enough to act on your behalf to make sure you get the best care possible. Let this person serve as your *advocate*, especially during those times when you are too tired or frustrated to be your own.

For me that someone was my wife, Jamie. For you it might be a spouse, a sibling, an adult child, or a best friend. Pick an advocate, and let that person in. Talk about your fears. Ask that person to accompany you to the hospital for the surgery and to be in the recovery room when you wake. Ask for help during the initial weeks of recovery, too.

But only tell other people about your heart disease on a need-to-know basis. We all have those people in our lives whose very presence does not allow us to feel strong, happy, and calm. Something about them rubs us the wrong way and causes us to feel tense. You definitely do not need such people visiting you while you are in the hospital, and you have the right to turn them away.

Most of us also know people who like to gossip and seem to enjoy spreading bad news about the hardships of others. You do not need people talking about you behind your back while you are recovering.

Finally, some of us work with people who are very competitive and who will use any sign of weakness as a personal advantage to get ahead in the work world. You do not need people using the details of your illness for their own personal gain.

For those reasons and more, I recommend that you do not announce your heart disease or upcoming operation. I often question my decision to have my bypass at the same hospital where I worked. That one decision broadcast my disease to everyone on staff and left me open to their gossip and backbiting. Tell the folks at work only what you must tell them in order to get sick leave and time off. To me, this is a very critical point.

Limit your "need to know" crowd to family and very, very close friends. Write the names of these people on a list, and give this list to the hospital floor nurse with detailed instructions that she or he should only allow people on the list to visit you. Will some visitors be disappointed when they learn they are not among the chosen few? Of course. Will some people feel slighted? Almost definitely. Right now, however, your health and personal sanity are much more important than the feelings of others who want to visit.

This is even true for family members. Some family members will not be able to deal with what is happening to you. When I had my bypass, my mother was eighty-eight. The idea that she might outlive me blew her mind. She did not come to the hospital, and that was good for both of us. Let family members know that you would prefer no visit to a tense one.

Take as much time off as you can. If you have disability insurance, look into activating it during your recovery time. Talk to the human resources department at work to find out how much vacation and sick leave you can take. Consider taking additional unpaid leave if you can afford to.

If your spouse works, see if she or he can take some time off, too, especially during the first few weeks of your recovery and longer if possible.

Pack the following things to take with you. You'll need a pair of slip-on shoes. You'll wear these during your trip back home postsurgery, as you won't be able to bend over to tie your shoelaces. Also pack a very comfortable outfit, one that is easy to get your arms in and out of. A bathrobe will do just fine! Consider taking a baseball cap and sunglasses, too,

❖ THE UNBEATABLES ❖

Joshua Lurie-Terrell didn't smoke. He weighed 187 pounds. He swam a mile several times a week and walked two miles every day. His cholesterol had always been below 180. He had only a small family history of heart disease. Then, at age thirty-seven, he suffered a mild heart attack. Here's how he came to grips with the question "Why me?"

When it happened, I was totally in shock. I could think of a hundred other people who were more likely to have a heart attack than I was. I could not believe it. My parents could not believe it. No one could believe it.

Once the initial shock wore off, however, I began to worry. My wife and I were two years into a quest to adopt a baby. I thought, "How can I hide this from the adoption agency so they won't refuse to give us a baby? If I do die, I need to do it after the baby gets here, so I won't let my wife down."

And then the depression set in. I worried, "What if I die tomorrow?" I felt like a crummy husband and father because my family would not be able to count on me to stick around. My mind swam with questions that had no answers: *How could I have gotten to the point that people could not rely on me? Why me? I don't deserve this, do I?* I felt like the universe was mad at me, and I could not figure out what I'd done to offend it.

My cardiologist really helped me. He was very hands-on. He called me every other day to make sure I was going to my cardiac rehabilitation class. I was the youngest person there! Most of the other guys there were twenty years older, much heavier, and a lot less fit. I thought, "If these guys can recover from this, so can I. I have a chance to fix this."

So I started riding my bike three miles each morning to get to rehab, where I would run a couple of miles and do free weights. Then I would ride home. I began taking medication to control my cholesterol, and I began eating differently—a lot differently.

Before my diagnosis, my friends called me "Bacon." I loved going to greasy spoon restaurants for burgers, BLTs, and other types of really fatty-red-meat meals. Now I've increased my consumption of seafood probably 300 percent, and I make sure I eat lots of raw vegetables every day. I eat carrots and broccoli at my desk, and lots of nuts, too. I also drink several cups of black or green tea. When I want to indulge, I do, but I do it in a healthy way with dark chocolate.

Do I miss all those fatty foods that I used to eat? Of course I do, but I think of it this way: What will I miss more, bacon or my family?

I feel more responsible for my mental and physical health now, too. I take more vacations. I stay home more with my daughter. I do more work that I like doing, and less that I don't. For instance, I'm less likely to spend time updating my Hewn and Hammered website and blog about crafts and design or to accept side freelance graphic design work. Instead I try to spend as much time as I can with my family. I'm more likely, for instance, to decide to go for a walk at night with my wife and daughter than I am to do any type of work or hobby.

As a result of all of these changes, I've lost twenty pounds. I've lowered my cholesterol, and my heart has recovered. My heart attack damaged the bottom of my heart muscle, but my most recent cardio-gram shows that most of my heart is healthy and functioning. Most of the damage has been eliminated.

Joshua's Unbeatable Advice: You cannot do this alone. If it wasn't for the other guys and the very supportive nurses in my cardiac rehabilita-tion class, I could not have done this. My wife tried to help me. My family tried to help me. But it was seeing those guys every day that allowed me to know that I was not alone. They understood what I was going through because they were going through it, too. That made a big difference.

especially if you'll be in the hospital for a few days. After being indoors that long, the glare of the sun can be uncomfortable, and you don't need any-thing else to make you even more uncomfortable during that long, hard walk from the hospital door to your waiting car. You also might want to bring a puffy jacket, such as a ski jacket. You'll wear it during discharge, not necessarily to keep you warm, but to protect your tender incision area and prevent other people from getting too close to you.

Also pack small items that you will find comforting to either look at or listen to as you recover. These items will vary from person to person and can include anything and everything from a music player to photo-graphs to a lucky charm.

The Stuff Only a Doctor Can Tell You

Just before and after surgery, there are several things that I suggest you request of the hospital staff. They include the following:

Ask to have your breathing tube removed while you are still

under. When you go under general anesthesia, a breathing tube is placed in your windpipe to ensure proper breathing during surgery. This is necessary and lifesaving, but not something you want to experience while you are fully conscious.

I've seen the looks of terror on people's faces when they wake and realize a machine is breathing for them. It's incredibly scary and unpleasant to have a breathing tube removed while you are conscious. Avoid it if possible by asking the medical staff to remove your tube while you are still sedated. Also, make sure, if you must be awake during the removal, that a loved one is in the room with you to hold your hand and offer encouragement and support during the process.

Ask to be given a sedative before surgery. There's no reason to feel terrified as they wheel you into the operating room. Ask for something to calm you beforehand. Your anesthesiologist should be able to give you something intravenously, such as Valium.

Ask if the hospital allows overnight visitors so a spouse or other loved one can stay with you in your room the entire night. Don't be macho about this. Don't say, "Oh, that's okay, get your rest." You are the one who needs your rest. Allow your caregiver to be there for you. There's nothing scarier than being alone in your room in the middle of the night and wondering just how long it will take a nurse to respond to you pressing the call button. If you are in a semiprivate room, your spouse or other loved one can sleep in a chair or even in a sleeping bag on the floor. If you upgrade to (and pay extra for) a private room, your loved one will have more space. I did and it was worth it.

Ask for sleeping medication. There's absolutely nothing wrong with taking a medication to help you sleep, especially during the first couple of nights after surgery. It's hard to sleep in a hospital, even when you are

The night before Marc's surgery, one of his colleagues stopped by his room to complain about a hospital policy that affected only his department. He started arguing with Marc. I sat there, staring at them both in disbelief. Here we were, the night before my husband was to undergo a surgery that could quite possibly kill him. We had many family matters to discuss, including what I would do about the mortgage if he didn't make it? What would I tell the kids if things didn't go well? How would I care for his aging mother? She lived in our neighborhood and had moved to New York to be closer to Marc because her own health was failing. He needed to tell me about his concerns regarding the surgery itself and how I could better be an advocate on his behalf while he was under anesthesia. I needed to talk about my fears, too, especially about possibly being left to care for his two children, my son, and his mother. It should have been a very personal time, one reserved just for family. Here was this guy bringing up a trivial work issue?!

I finally said, "Look, you are going to have to leave," and he did.

You may have to do the same. It might be neighbors or extended family or coworkers. It could be anyone, even someone who means well. It might even be one of your kids! It doesn't matter. The night before surgery and just after surgery are not times for lots of visitors. Keep visits with children to just ten minutes at a time, and put a DO NOT DISTURB sign on the door. Ask the nursing staff to ask visitors to return at a later date.

pain free. Hospital staff will wake you repeatedly as they fiddle with catheters, blood pressure cuffs, and monitoring devices. Most hospital personnel truly don't care whether or not you get any sleep. They just want to make sure that the surgery took and that your heart muscle is getting enough blood flow. Sleep medicine will help you sleep through all this, so you can heal more quickly. For a detailed description of specific sleep medicines, see Chapter 3.

When they are removing your catheter after surgery, ask whether or not it is deflated. Occasionally nurses forget to deflate urinary catheters before removing them. When this happens, it's incredibly painful. I know, because it happened to me! I bled from the damage. If this can happen to the person who runs the surgical department at the very hospital where the procedure is performed, it can happen to anyone!

From Hospital to Home

You'll be in the hospital anywhere from one day (for a stent) to three days or longer for a bypass or heart attack. No matter the type of procedure or the length of stay, your trip home just might be one of the hardest and longest trips of your life. Here's what to do.

Wear slip-on shoes. Remember those slip-on shoes I suggested you pack? You'll need them for the trip home. Same with that comfortable outfit. Same with that baseball cap. Same with that puffy jacket.

Go with two people. Arrange to have someone pick you up at the hospital. Ideally, have one person drive and a passenger who can assist you, if needed, during the trip. Ask to be driven in the biggest car available, such as a van or station wagon. That way you can lie down if you feel you need to.

Go straight home. Don't stop to fill prescriptions or get anything from the store. A loved one or a friend can run out and get whatever you need later after getting you settled at home.

Before I left to pick Marc up from the hospital, I made a special effort to make our apartment seem as warm and inviting as possible. I made up the couch for Marc, so it would be ready for him to sit on as soon as he walked in the door. I had pillows and blankets stacked nearby, should he need them. I had soft music playing and I left the lights on. I wanted him to feel as if he was walking into a sanctuary.

Then, when we did walk in the door, I got him settled on the couch and I left him alone for a while. I knew he needed some time alone to cry, and that's what he did.

Your Emotional Wounds

Your physical wounds will heal in a matter of weeks. Your mental wounds will take much longer. You will ask, "Why me? Why did this happen to me? What did I do to deserve this?" You will tell yourself, "I am not strong enough to face this. I cannot go on. This is too hard."

You will worry, "What if I die? How will my family cope?"

You will experience any or all of the following:

Fear. You will come to grips with your mortality and what the inevitable end of your life—today, tomorrow, next year, next decade—means for the rest of your life. You now realize that the runway of life is continually getting shorter, that it doesn't go on forever, and that you are now probably closer to its end than you are to its beginning.

Remind yourself: "I'm still here. I'm still alive, and I'm going to make the best of it by facing down my fear and living the rest of my life to the fullest."

Guilt. You might blame yourself for ending up here. You might spend time obsessing about what you might have done wrong, analyzing your past diet, exercise habits, or stress level.

Remind yourself: "The past is the past. I can't change how I lived in the past. I can only change how I live today, and today I am doing all I can to beat heart disease."

Anger. You might have "Why Me Syndrome." For instance, you might tell yourself, "This isn't fair. I've had a healthy diet, have been very fit, and have never smoked. Why did I get heart disease while that overweight couch potato smokestack at work is completely healthy? It's not fair!"

Remind yourself: "Life isn't fair. There's nothing I can do about that right now. I can, however, focus on doing everything I can to get and stay better. I will live healthy to stay healthy."

Denial. You may, in the future, be tempted to tell yourself, "My surgery fixed me. I don't need to eat differently, de-stress, or exercise." The truth of the matter is that it only fixed you temporarily. If you do not do all you can to keep your arteries clear, they will indeed clog up again.

I'm willing to bet that you don't want to spend your last years on this earth confined to a bed. I'm willing to bet you don't want to spend your last years dependent on the help of others. I'm willing to bet you don't want to spend those years wishing you felt more energetic, less uncomfortable, and more mentally alert. Indeed, you want to die feeling healthy and fit. You want to age with strength and vitality. We all do.

Remind yourself: "Yes, my surgery bought me extra time. I want that time to last as long as possible, so I am going to do everything I can to get and stay better."

Loathing. You might come to loathe your body, both for how it looks (emaciated) and how it feels (achy, painful, and weak). You might come to loathe your mind, for inflicting the fear that keeps you from relaxing or for causing your thinking to seem clouded. I wish I could promise you that you would regain every aspect of your mental and physical capabilities after surgery. I can't. Some things just won't come back. You may have many losses.

- The loss of your body and how it once looked.
- The loss of what your body can do for you on any given day.
- The loss of your place in the hierarchy in the community or at work.
- The loss of your confidence.
- The loss of your naiveté about life and death.

Remind yourself: "I still want to live, despite my losses. I will define my life and I will learn from this. My heart disease will change me for the better."

Your Back-to-Life Plan

You can live your life again. You can experience yet another chapter in your book of life. Just follow in my footsteps.

No one is the same after this, but many people are better. You need to see this not as a death, but as a rebirth, as a chance to reinvent yourself for the better. As you ready yourself to embark on this important journey, I'd like you to think about two important questions.

Question #1: How do I want to die?

I suppose if we all had our way, we just wouldn't die. We would live forever. I wish I could promise that. Think of how many billions of books I could sell if I had the answer to eternal life!

I don't have that answer. No one does. We all die. Now that you've accepted this fact as an inevitable part of life, let's figure out what to do about it. Make a decision. How do you want to die? Personally, I want to die when I'm well into my eighties or nineties, when I'm running my twentieth or thirtieth or fortieth marathon. When I die, I want to feel healthy and strong. I want to feel at peace with the world. I want to die knowing that

I made the world a better place, that I was kind to people who needed my kindness. I want to die knowing that someone loves me.

That's how I want to go out.

So take some time right now to think about this question. Write down your answer and keep it handy. Use it as your motivation to do everything you can to live and keep living.

Question #2: How do I want to live?

What are your dreams? How do you want to be remembered? How do you want to make a difference? The answers to those questions just might give you the will to keep going when your recovery becomes tough and, believe me, it will get very tough.

Love of family can get you so far. Love of career can help, too.

Love of life? That's what gets you to the finish line.

❀   **BACK TO LIFE R$_x$**   ❀

- Get an advocate. Use as often as needed to supplement energy, courage, and assertiveness. Take with plenty of hand-holding, love, and understanding.
- When in doubt, seek second, third, and fourth opinions.
- Choose your doctor and hospital carefully, using health-care report cards and referrals from other patients and doctors.
- Put yourself first in the days before and after surgery. You don't have to be social. Turn away visitors if you need your rest or privacy.

❖ PART TWO ❖

The Plan

3

Step 1:
Conquer the Night

I WAS HIGHLY SEDATED MY FIRST NIGHT AT THE HOSPITAL. I REMEM-
ber little to nothing about it.

It wasn't until my second night that my fear of sleep set in. On this
night, I closed my eyes, turned to one side, and heard the familiar ba-
bump, ba-bump of my heart. I opened my eyes. My palms began to sweat.
I felt nauseous. My heart raced. It was as if I had woken to the image of
Jack the Ripper, standing over me with a knife. It was just my heart beating,
normally, but I was filled with fear.

Will I wake? Will I wake? Will I wake?

The physician in me knew I needed sleep. I knew that I needed at least
seven hours of shut-eye for my chest, breastbone, and vessels to heal from
the trauma of surgery. Yet I couldn't find the courage to close my eyes.

Every time I closed my eyes, I felt as if I was losing control. I worried that I would not wake again.

This went on night after night after night, starting at the hospital and continuing as I recuperated at home.

Fear of the Familiar

In surveys, the majority of bypass surgery patients complain of sleep problems initially and, for nearly half of patients, these problems persist for at least eight weeks.[1] Even while asleep, most surgical patients do not sleep deeply enough, with the rapid-eye-movement and delta-sleep stages either not happening at all or not happening as often as usual.

Yet sleep is important. Surgical patients who sleep better tend to recover more quickly physically and emotionally, and lack of sleep raises your risk of developing and worsening heart disease.[2,3]

Your first couple of nights probably will be your most difficult. For me, night #2 was worse than night #1. That's when everything hit me and I began to worry.

What is really going to happen to me? I am not ready for the junk heap. Will I ever be in control of my life again?

My fear of the night continued for a very long time. I eventually learned a number of strategies that could allow me to relax and feel calm at night. I've included those strategies—ranging from sleeping with the blinds open to using a sound machine—throughout this chapter. It wasn't until I started seeing a psychiatrist and got a prescription for sleeping pills, however, that I was finally able to sleep all night without waking up.

I used those pills for the first three months. Then I was able to sleep most nights without them. I still occasionally take one whenever I'm in a new environment, such as a hotel. If you need sleep medicine, as I did, there's nothing to feel embarrassed about. It's normal.

And it's important. That's why I've included it as the first tip in this chapter.

Throughout this chapter, you'll find what helped me get through those initial scary nights. Try it. I believe it will help you, too.

Talk to Your Cardiologist About the Best Sleep Medicine for You

You need sleep. It's important. If you can't sleep, you need a medicine to help, at least for the time being. Below you'll find a brief review of the most common sleep medicines. Remember to talk with your doctor before taking any medication, even if it's available over the counter.

Over-the-Counter Options

Diphenhydramine. This antihistamine, found in Nytol, Sominex, and a few other brands, helps induce sleep by countering the effects of histamine, a chemical messenger that promotes wakefulness. Benadryl also induces sleepiness the same way. These products are all available over the counter. Talk to your cardiologist about whether they are right for you.

Doxylamine. This is another antihistamine, found in brands like Unisom.

Melatonin. Melatonin is a sleep-inducing hormone. No research, however, supports the effectiveness of supplemental melatonin for inducing sleep in insomniacs, and this over-the-counter option probably is not strong enough to help induce sleep after surgery.

You might realize that your heartbeat is more noticeable after bypass surgery or angioplasty. This is a good thing! Your heart is beating more strongly thanks to all of that new blood flow.

You'll probably be most aware of the sound of your heart more at night as you lie in bed. The truth of the matter is that your heart is always beating, with roughly the same cadence and volume, all day long. You don't hear it because you are distracted by the other noises around you, such as traffic, conversations, and the television. When you lie down and the distractions stop, you are suddenly able to hear your heart. If the sound of your heart makes you anxious, lie on your back. It won't be as noticeable.

Herbs. Many herbs are thought to improve sleep. They include chamomile, valerian root, kava kava, lemon balm, and lavender, among others. I often drink chamomile tea in the evenings and find it relaxing and comforting.

Prescription Options

Prescription options generally are more effective than what you can find over the counter, but some can worsen depression. If you suffer from postsurgical depression, and many post-op cardiac patients do (see Chapter 4), work closely with your doctor to find the best sleeping medicine and antidepressant combination for you.

Dalmane, Doral, Restoril, and other benzodiazepine sedatives. This is the oldest class of sleeping pills and is considered the most habit-forming. These pills may also worsen depression.

Lunesta, Ambien, Sonata, and other non-benzodiazepine sedatives. This newer class of sleeping pills acts more selectively in the brain and may have fewer side effects and less risk of addiction than its older cousins. Do not combine them with alcohol, and take them only before you plan to sleep for at least seven or eight hours.

Rozerem. This prescription sleep aid helps regulate the sleep hormone melatonin. It's milder than other sleeping pills, but also less habit-forming. Like other prescription sleep aids, it may worsen depression.

Take pain medication a half hour before bedtime. This ensures that you will be pain free most of the night. I also got in the habit of keeping a pain pill and glass of water on my nightstand, so I could wake, take my medication (if needed), and go right back to sleep.

Say the following over and over again. "I will wake up. I will wake up." Your first or second night will be the most difficult, and then every night after that will become easier. Remind yourself that your surgery fixed your heart. Remember that you are more likely to wake tomorrow than you were yesterday. In fact, you faced a much higher likelihood of dying in your sleep last night than you do tonight.

Once you get through the first night, remind yourself that you got through last night, so you will get through this night, too. Say, "I was successful the first night after surgery. If I could fall asleep *that* night and wake the next day, I can fall asleep *any* night."

Train for Better Sleep

What you do during the day will affect how well you sleep at night. Try the following:

Go back to bed after breakfast. I didn't fear the bed during the day as I did at night, so I used the morning and midafternoon for sleep training. When you wake in the morning, get out of bed, do your morning routine, and have breakfast. Then pretend it's nighttime. Go through the motions of going to sleep. Stay in your pajamas, brush your teeth, and do everything else you usually do before going to bed. Then get into bed. Just lie there and relax for thirty to sixty minutes. This will help break your association of the bed with your fear of dying. I still do this occasionally on mornings when I have the extra time.

You may not have had a bedtime routine before surgery, but you'll probably need one now. Do the following:

Take a hot bath before bed. For years I've told my patients that wet heat or warm water helps them heal, and relieves incision discomfort. Now I know it is true! A hot bath takes you to the womb, helping you relax and forget about all those worries that are keeping you awake. The heat on the incision also reduces discomfort, and encourages circulation, which will help you heal.

Most important, the bath will raise your body temperature, which has been shown to enhance stage 3 and 4 sleep, the non-rapid-eye-movement stages that are most restorative for the body.[4]

In a Japanese study, nine women took a hot bath, immersed their legs (up to their knees) in a hot footbath, or did neither before bedtime. When the women took a bath or used the footbath, they fell asleep more quickly and slept more deeply than when they did neither before bed. They also tossed and turned less often.[5]

Use this advice:

- Use a footbath for the initial days after surgery, until your physician gives you the okay to submerge your incision in water. You can usually immerse your wound in water around the fourth day post-surgery.
- Take care getting in and out of the tub. Jamie had to help me, which wasn't fun for either of us. Here I was feeling less than sexy with my emaciated body. I had fallen into this depression and now I had to ask this beautiful woman to help me get in and out of the tub! I felt terrible about it, but I knew it was necessary. The last thing I

> needed was to slip and fall. If my incision had popped open from a
> fall, it would have put me in the hospital for one to three weeks.
> - Avoid showers before bed. They are too probing, not to mention
>   difficult in the very beginning.
> - Stay in the tub or use the footbath for at least a half hour.
> - Use a warm to hot temperature of 100° to 104°F.
> - If you use a footbath instead of a tub, make sure the container is
>   large enough for you to immerse your legs up to your knees.

Lie down midday, too. Do some more sleep training. Even take a nap if you feel tired. You'll need the extra sleep during the initial weeks after surgery anyway. Don't force yourself to sleep, however, if you are not tired. That's not the point. Just lie there and relax calmly for a half hour, and then get up. This again will help you associate sleep with comfort and calm rather than fear. Moreover, for me, it was a form of meditation.

Start a fitness program as soon as you can. The fitter and healthier you are, the more you will be able to believe that your heart is strong and healthy. The more you believe that your heart is strong and healthy, the less you will worry about dying in your sleep. The faster your heart beats during exercise, the more you will know that it will keep beating through the night. Use the cardiac rehabilitation program offered by your hospital as a kickoff for your fitness program. Once you graduate from cardiac rehabilitation, continue to exercise and stay in shape. Not only will it take the fear out of getting to sleep, it will help you sleep more deeply, too. Exercise in any form is wonderful for self-confidence as you recover.

It's so easy to focus on what you can't do early in your recovery. Try, instead, to notice what you can do. If you manage to take a nap without worry, that's great! If you get to sleep at all, you're moving in the right direction. You got yourself back to sleep at night after waking? Celebrate that morning with a Coffee Float (see recipe, page 250). When you take the time to notice every small change for the better, you'll feel more hopeful about your overall recovery.

Drink some warm milk. This folk remedy might help induce sleep because it contains the amino acid tryptophan, which the brain converts to the calming chemical serotonin, needed for healthy sleep.

Snuggle or sleep with a pet. Pets offer unconditional love, which is so important postsurgery when your self-esteem may be at its lowest point. They don't judge. They just love you, no matter what.

It's probably for this reason that studies show that snuggling with a beloved pet can help reduce levels of the stress hormone cortisol, which may very well help you get to sleep.[6] More important, research on more than 1,000 people done at the University of California at San Diego found that pet owners had lower blood pressure. A different study of more than 4,300 people determined that owning a cat reduced heart attack risk by a third.

Don't sleep with a pet, however, if your dog or cat tends to move around a lot at night. That might disturb your sleep more than it will help. Instead, try snuggling for a while before bed and then have your pet sleep somewhere else, unless their touch comforts you spiritually. Believe me, you will know.

Relax before bed. In the hour before bed, spend time doing relaxing activities. Take a bath. Read. Listen to soft music.

Breathe deeply. When you lie down at night, spend some time focusing on your breathing. This will help you relax. Inhale deeply, so your abdomen and rib cage expand with the breath. Exhale gently, feeling your entire body relax and compress. Do this over and over until you feel relaxed and sleepy.

Your Sleep Environment

A few changes to your bedroom environment can help you sleep more soundly.

Leave the shades or blinds open. During those initial fearful nights, I could not sleep in a dark room. If I woke to darkness, I would think, "Have I died?" I needed the light from a streetlight shining through my window to remind me that I was indeed alive and there was life outside. Similarly, weather permitting, I liked to leave the window open a crack so I could hear the sounds from outside—passing cars, garbage trucks, and general night life. It helped to convince myself that I could indeed live through this.

Use a night-light. This works in the same way as does leaving the shades open.

Take a familiar object to bed with you. It might be a pet, a heavy blanket, or something that represents your ability to heal and grow stronger.

Consider a sound machine. They are calming and can help soothe you to sleep. Most machines offer several options, ranging from white noise to rain to waves. I still use one to lull myself to sleep at home, and I have a smaller one that I take with me when I travel.

Adjust the room temperature or use extra blankets. After surgery, you'll probably find that you are colder than usual. This chill is often induced by sadness and depression. If you have little to no appetite, it can also stem from lack of food, as the metabolism of food tends to heat the body. No matter the reason, the sensation of warmth takes you back to the womb, which helps you relax and heal. There are few problems you can't overcome in a warm environment.

So add extra blankets on your side of the bed, especially heavy ones, as heaviness also tends to induce relaxation. In addition to keeping you warm, they will make you feel safe and secure. I still do this, and it really works for me.

Investigate your bedroom environment. Make sure none of the common factors that tend to wake people—even people without heart disease—are present in your bedroom. These include:

- Uncomfortable bedding or pillows. It's critical for your bed to be a warm and inviting place.
- Noise (a snoring spouse, a pet who whines or walks around, a clock ticking, a television set blasting sound in another room). Note that you might find some noise comforting—soft music on the radio or the TV on very low volume—because these sounds will remind you that you are still alive and not alone if you happen to wake in the middle of the night.
- Too much light, but not pitch-black.

When Fear Strikes in the Middle of the Night

Despite the best of daytime and bedtime routines, you may still find yourself lying awake with worry. Try this advice.

Talk to yourself. For me the night was when the obsessive questioning started. I would wonder: Will I be able to go back to work? Will I be able to support my family? Will I see my children age? What would happen to my mother if I died before she did? Will I be able to make love to my wife again? Will I be able to resume a normal life again?

When you find yourself overcome with these obsessive fears, do two things. First, talk about them. Ask your spouse to validate you and remind you that, yes, of course you will be able to do all of those things once you recover. (Note that your children may not be the best people to share these fears with, because they have so many fears of their own about what life would be like without you.)

Second, do everything you can to remind yourself that you are alive. I used to lie on my back and place my hand on the side of my neck just below my jawbone so I could feel my pulse. I would then take deep breaths. As I did so, I told myself over and over: *Your heart is beating. Your heart is beating. Your heart is beating. You must be okay. Your heart is beating.* It became my mantra.

Other soothing mantras include:

You are alive. Yes, you could have died, but now you are alive. Your life has been spared.

God spared you. You have a second chance at living. You've been given a next chapter.

I have a lot to accomplish, to love my wife, take care of my patients [insert something specific to your profession here], see my children and grandchildren grow and mature, which gives my life so much meaning.

Promise to wake up. At first, sleeping for a full seven or eight hours can seem overwhelming. So break sleep into chunks. For instance, during my initial nights after surgery, I promised myself that I would wake at 2 or 3 a.m. As I fell asleep, I put it in my mind that I would wake in the middle of the night, check and make sure I was still alive, and then go back to sleep. It may sound silly, but I found it incredibly reassuring. I would wake at 2 or 3, hear my heart beating, and tell myself, "I'm still here." Then I would go back to sleep feeling more relaxed.

Get up and take your mind off things. If you lie awake for more than a half hour, get out of bed. Do something to take your mind off your thoughts. Get a glass of water or make some herbal (noncaffeinated) tea with milk. Chamomile works for me. Walk around. Look out a window. Remind yourself that these worries are just your mind playing tricks on you. You are fine. See, you are walking around! You are looking out a window! You are going to be okay. Then, once you feel sleepy and relaxed, go back to bed.

Do everything you can to convince yourself that your procedure was done well. If needed, schedule an extra appointment with your cardiologist. Talk about the worries that are keeping you awake at night. For instance, tell your cardiologist that you are worried that you will not recover physically. Then your cardiologist can tell you exactly what to expect and when. Similarly, if you are worried about having a heart attack, your cardiologist can show you just how strong your heart is now.

Your cardiologist can do an echocardiogram, for instance, to show you that your heart is still beating (see Chapter 6 for more on how tests can help you heal). The right cardiologist will understand your issues.

It will take a while but, eventually, you'll find that you just stop thinking about going to sleep and whether or not you will wake up. Sleep eventually will become habitual for you again.

And then, just like that, it won't. This probably will happen when you have to sleep in new surroundings. For me it happened during my first business trip, about six months after my bypass, when I slept in a hotel out of town. I was away from all the comforts of home. I didn't have my sound machine. I didn't have Jamie. I didn't have Mady, our four-pound Yorkshire terrier!

I've since learned to take as much "home" with me as possible when I travel. I can't always take Jamie, but I can and do take the sound machine. I sometimes even take Mady. I just make sure to stay in pet-friendly hotels and I ignore the part of myself that is embarrassed by the stares of other people who see me carrying this little dog in a dog carrier. Hey, at least I can sleep at night!

I also leave the blinds open, so I can see light at night if I wake. I try to book a room with a view, too, so I have something to look at if I wake at night and find myself standing at the window.

It's still a little harder to sleep when I travel, but it's not impossible. I can sleep at night. You can, too.

4

Step 2:
Face Physical and
Emotional Pain

BEFORE BYPASS SURGERY, THE STRONGEST PAIN MEDICATION I EVER took was Darvocet, a prescription-strength Tylenol with codeine. It didn't come close to preparing me for the experience of taking OxyContin, a narcotic pain reliever that works like morphine. Despite strong FDA warnings about the potential addictiveness of this pain reliever, it's still one of the most prescribed pain medicines for heart surgery patients.[1]

Boy, does it take away the pain—all of the pain. During the initial week after surgery, I really did need the narcotic. My surgeon had sliced through the center of my chest—all the way through my sternum—to get access to the blood vessels surrounding my heart. Once he bypassed my arteries, he wired my breastbone back together. It would take six or so weeks for the bone to grow back together, and even longer for the surrounding muscle and other tissues to recover.

As a result, every time I moved, it hurt! It would have hurt when I was sitting still, too, had I not been on painkillers.

But the painkillers took away the pain. They did a very good job of that, almost too good a job.

The problem was that each twice-daily dose not only took away my chest pain, it also removed my emotional pain. It made me high, and lifted my severe postoperative depression.

If it weren't for Jamie, I'd probably still be taking the stuff. I probably should have been on strong painkillers like OxyContin for just a few days. After just three days I could have switched to something less addictive such as Vicodin, Tylenol with Codeine, or Percocet. I had many, many options.

But I didn't use them. On day eight I was still taking OxyContin. I told myself I needed it for the pain, but Jamie knew better.

Jamie saw me take two OxyContins and asked, "Are you in pain?" I replied, "Not right now! Right now, I have no pain at all." She said sarcastically, "I bet you don't. This has got to stop." She gathered up the rest of my pain meds and flushed them down the toilet. I watched, and I cried.

Eventually, however, I realized that I was depressed and needed help. I started seeing a therapist and taking antidepressants. I also tried the advice you will find in this chapter.

How to Avoid Addiction

Prescription painkillers such as OxyContin can reduce anxiety and generate a sensation of euphoria. If you take them for more than a few days or abuse them and take too much, you will go through a period of withdrawal that will make you feel restless, anxious, irritable, and sick (sweaty, chilly, and nauseous). The withdrawal can even trigger physical pain, which will cause you to believe that you really did need the painkillers in the first place.

As a result, somewhere between 10 and 40 percent of people who take prescription painkillers become addicted to them. Anxiety, depression, and loneliness—all very common feelings postsurgery—increase the likelihood of addiction. You might be addicted to your pain meds if any of the following are true:

- You use more medicine than you've been prescribed.
- You go to multiple doctors so you can get multiple prescriptions of the same painkiller.
- You use alcohol and other medicines to increase the high you feel from the painkillers.
- You take painkillers when you are not physically uncomfortable.
- You take painkillers to soothe anxiety or stress.
- Your spouse and other loved ones are worried about your use of pain medication.

To prevent addiction, use this advice:

Ask your partner or other loved one to control your meds. Your partner should ask you to rate your pain on a scale of 1 to 10, with 10 being the most excruciating pain you have ever experienced in your life and 1 being bliss. To receive meds, your pain should be between 7 and 10. If it's between 3 and 6, you probably can get by with over-the-counter medicines such as Extra Strength Tylenol or aspirin. If you rank your pain as low as 1 or 2, you may not need to take anything.

In lieu of pain medicine, try the following natural pain-soothing strategies.

- Take a warm bath. The warm water increases blood flow to your wound, speeding healing and calming discomfort. To boost your mood, use scented bubble bath and light candles.
- Go for a walk. It will help reduce anxiety and boost your mood, helping you see that the "pain" was emotional and not physical. Make sure to walk during the day, so you can both see where you are going and benefit from the mood-boosting effects of sunlight. Sunlight helps lighten your mood. Plus, going for a walk allows you to see other people and lets you know that you are among the living.
- Watch something engaging on TV. It might be sports, a cooking show, a documentary, or a movie. It will take your mind off the discomfort.
- Listen to music. You will lose yourself in the music and temporarily forget about the pain.[2] Research done at South Dakota State University on sixty-one patients recovering from open-heart surgery determined that those who listened to thirty minutes of music were less anxious and experienced less pain than patients who did not listen to music.[3,4,5] Interestingly, the music that you find most helpful may not necessarily be the music you liked to listen to before your diagnosis. I grew up in Philadelphia and was a rhythm and blues fan. I even enjoyed hip-hop; I played it in the operating room! After my surgery, however, I could only listen to classical music. Mozart, Beethoven, and Brahms soothed me at home and in the car. (Now that I've fully recovered, though, I'm back to my old standbys!)

❖ THE UNBEATABLES ❖

Bill Wohl, a former collegiate and professional athlete, was a successful businessman who designed electronics systems for sports arenas and home theaters, hobnobbed with top sports idols, and earned a seven-figure income. Then, at age fifty-two, the big one hit. His heart was starving for oxygen, its cells suffocating and dying, but he didn't go to the hospital. He thought he was suffering from food poisoning. It wasn't until seven hours after experiencing chest pain that he called 911. At the hospital, he got the news that no one wants to hear. He'd suffered a heart attack. His heart muscle was destroyed. He had congestive heart failure.

Next, his liver, kidneys, and lungs began to fail, too. Wohl needed a transplant, but a new heart was not yet available and he was too sick to make the transplant list. Doctors implanted an experimental artificial heart, called the CardioWest temporary Total Artificial Heart, instead. Nearly half a year later, he got a donor heart. Now, nine years later, he's winning triathlons and cycling, swimming, and track events. Here's how he made his comeback.

———

I went from fit former college athlete to a successful but fat businessman. I thought my life was perfect, too. What could be better than to make a lot of money, build a big house, and deal with half the people at ESPN SportsCenter on a regular basis? What kid doesn't dream of growing up and having a client list that reads like a Who's Who Among American Athletes? When the owner of the Chicago Bulls and White Sox called me one day and suggested that I go to Michael Jordan's house to do some electronics work, I couldn't have been happier.

But it all came at a price. I did a great job taking care of my wife and my clients, but I didn't do a great job taking care of myself. My doctors think my heart problems can be traced primarily to my negligence in getting dental care! In the year before my heart attack, I had a huge jaw infection that I was unaware of. The bacteria from that infection invaded my bloodstream, causing the plaque that led to two 100 percent blockages and a heart attack. I didn't address that problem until after the heart attack. As if I didn't have enough to worry about with my heart, I had to undergo a root canal that year, too!

I almost died in the hospital many times. At one point, I was in a coma for a full month. Many people who were much fitter and healthier than I have died from much less severe blockages and heart damage. I shouldn't have survived two 100 percent blockages for as long as I did. Several doctors have told me that.

Soon after my release from the hospital, I saw a video about the U.S. Transplant Games. I'd swum and cycled when I was a kid, and I ran track when I was in high school and college. I decided to start training. Two years later, I competed in the U.S. Transplant Games, winning two silvers.

I've been training for something ever since. I compete almost monthly in some type of open competition. It's now nine years and twenty-three individual and five relay gold medals in National Transplant Games Championships later. I've competed in the United States, Canada, Australia, France, and Thailand.

Before my heart attack, I'd loved my job. Who wouldn't? I got to interact with the top sports stars and coaches in the country! But I also worked nearly nonstop, and was always on call. Now I feel really blessed that my heart problems taught me that work is not the most important thing in my life. Being happy and healthy is.

I still work, but a lot less, and I spend my nonworking hours getting myself in shape for whatever race I happen to be training for and building my nonprofit Bill Wohl Foundation, which is a donor-awareness center.

Bill's Unbeatable Advice: You are on the bad side right now. Eat, sleep, breathe, and dream of the good side. Look at what you really would like to do and where you would like to go. Who would you like to be? Then find a way to chase your dream and begin living it.

Keep a pain medication log. That way both you and your doctor can see how often you need and take pain meds. The log may help you see that you are taking more than you really need. In the log, write down how much and how often you took pain medicines, as well as your 1 to 10 pain rankings, and bring it to all medical appointments.

Consider acupuncture. Various studies show that acupuncture can help reduce physical pain, with relief lasting three to six months.[6] In one study on people with back pain, acupuncture was twice as effective as pain medication![7]

Face Emotional Pain

Right after surgery I went into a funk. I worried constantly—about whether I would be able to go back to work and support my family, pay the mortgage, and make love to my wife again. I dreamed about what would have happened had I not stopped running in Central Park the day that I noticed the chest pain. What if I had kept going instead of turning back? In my dreams I collapsed in Central Park and did not get back up. I died. I lost many nights' sleep over these dreams!

The painkillers initially took these worries away—along with my fear of my own mortality. Once Jamie flushed those pain meds down the toilet, however, I needed to find a way to come to terms with the new me, my new life, and my new limitations.

It's important for you to do the same. A startling percentage of heart attack and heart surgery survivors don't make comebacks. Their hearts are still beating. They are technically alive. Yet they've died emotionally.

Consider:

- Nearly one in three heart attack survivors becomes depressed, a condition that doubles their risk of death. Among people with heart disease who have not suffered an attack, the statistic is one in five. That makes depression four times more common among people with heart disease than the general population. Feelings of helplessness, fear, and anxiety are also common.
- In a study of nine hundred heart attack survivors, nearly all survivors under age sixty-five continued to report reduced quality of life a full four years after their initial attack.
- A Harris Interactive survey of more than five hundred heart attack survivors determined that most survivors fear another attack more than death, yet 40 percent admit that they are not doing all they can to stay healthy.

In retrospect I realize that I was experiencing the same emotions that many of the cancer survivors I'd treated had told me about over the years. Their physical symptoms were different. Instead of the racing heartbeat, they felt phantom pain in their back, head, hips—any part of the body where they worried the cancer might return. These phantom physical symptoms are one of the hallmarks of post-traumatic stress disorder (PTSD). Although PTSD has been associated with war veterans and rape survivors, it is also very common in survivors of major illness. Symptoms include re-experiencing the initial trauma through flashbacks or nightmares; avoiding certain people, places, activities, or other reminders of the health trauma; and a faster and more easily triggered startle reflex. This may result in trouble sleeping or concentrating.

PTSD and depression are troubling because they not only prevent you from living life again, but also can become a self-fulfilling prophecy. Research has found that the emotional stress created by PTSD and depression can worsen heart disease. Depression, for instance, increases your risk of heart trouble by increasing low-grade inflammation, which, in turn, leads to artery clogging. It activates platelets, too, making them more sticky and more likely to clump together into deadly blood clots. It alters the rhythm of your heartbeat and increases your blood pressure, insulin, cholesterol, and stress hormone levels. Leave it untreated and your risk of death during the next four months is four times higher than someone with heart disease who is not depressed. It also makes you less likely to practice all the other things you know you should be doing—eating right, exercising, and refraining from smoking, just to name a few.

You will go through a stage of grief and sadness. That's normal. You may not want to be dependent. Your self-esteem may be shot. You may feel guilty or frustrated about your past (what led to your diagnosis). And you may feel anxious about the future.

How do you know if you are experiencing normal sadness or depression that should be treated? You may be depressed if you have two or more of the following symptoms:

- Lack of appetite
- Prolonged sadness or weepiness
- Insomnia
- Irritability or anger
- Lethargy
- Difficulty concentrating
- Constipation
- Lack of interest in getting dressed
- Avoiding interaction with others, especially outside the house
- Feeling lost or helpless
- Feeling as if life is no longer worth living
- Thoughts of death or suicide

Depression is more than just a temporary sadness. It affects every part of your life. It takes away the pleasure of eating, sleeping, and living. It can even make you feel tired and sore.

As your loved one grieves, provide healthy doses of comedic relief whenever possible. Don't make light of his or her situation, but certainly don't avoid the discussion of amusing events when they arise. For example, I took time off from work while Marc was recovering but, after four weeks, I knew I needed to get a new job closer to home. So I started interviewing.

I went to an interview at a local television station that I knew very little about. I wore a pants suit with a camisole that day. I thought I looked professional and attractive.

When I walked into the interviewer's office, my potential employer said, "Who told you I was a boob man? I'm into legs."

I thought, "I obviously can never work for this man. I might as well have a little fun."

"By the way," he continued, "you should see the hottie I just hired. She used to be a trainer."

I nonchalantly said, "Oh, yeah? I bet I can take her. Why don't you bring her in?" When he looked up at me, I could see in his eyes that he was envisioning a female fight to the finish. He could not get out of his chair fast enough and rushed out of his office to find this female reporter. I could not believe that he thought I was serious.

He walked back into the office. He was out of breath and dejected, saying, "I couldn't find her."

I said, "That's okay, because this fight would be a Gold Card Event."

At that remark, he threw all of his credit cards on the table.

I knew it was time to go.

As I walked back home, I cried. I really needed that job. Then, when

I opened the door and saw Marc sitting on the couch, I thought, "I have nothing to cry about." I started laughing, hysterically.

When Marc asked me whether I got the job, I laughed even more. Then I told him about the comment about "not being a boob man" and the proposed female wrestling match, and it was his turn to laugh. He laughed so hard. It was the first time I'd seen him laugh that much since before his surgery.

From then on, I made a point of trying to get him to laugh. I bought him Jackie Mason DVDs and CDs and joke books. And I made sure to keep a king-size pillow nearby, so he could hug it to his chest to stifle the pain from his incision caused by his laughter. Laughter really helped him recover.

Here's the thing with depression: It goes hand in hand with denial. In eight weeks, I'd lost twenty pounds due to lack of appetite. None of my clothes fit, but when I looked in the mirror, I thought I looked normal. My depression tried to convince me that my ineffective coping mechanisms were beneficial. It tried to trick me into thinking that I was fine, that I didn't need help.

But I did need help.

Depression is very common, but it's not something you should live with. To release yourself from the past and embrace a better future, use this advice.

Give yourself time to mourn. Cry. Beat your fists on the table. Get the anger, frustration, and sadness out. Don't bury it. Face it and ponder it. This will take tremendous strength. You may need your partner or a therapist to help you through it.

Stop asking, "Why me?" Instead ask, "What could be?" When you ask, "Why me?" or "Why did this happen to me?" you live in the past, in a time and dimension you cannot control. It may not be fair that you had a heart attack, needed stents, or needed surgery. Maybe you did everything right. I know I did. I ran marathons. I followed a healthful diet. I was also under a lot of stress and had a strong genetic history of heart disease. I realize now that trying to change the past was futile. I couldn't change my genetics. I couldn't change the fact that I lived on fast food when I was a teenager and young adult. I couldn't change the fact that I had a very stressful job. I *could* change the future. I knew I needed to modify my life and lifestyle, but I also knew I needed to do it slowly and incrementally.

Get dressed every day, even if you don't plan to go outdoors. The act of getting dressed says, "I am alive and I am going to actively participate in the rest of my life."

Walk every day, preferably outside. The sunlight, social interaction of saying "hello," or smiling at the people you pass, and the exercise will all help calm you and improve your outlook on life.

Admit it. Tell your loved one or doctor how you feel. Sometimes the simple act of saying "I need help" can be liberating. Plus your loved one and doctor can help you get the treatment you need. Your doctor can help you decide if you need antidepressant medication to help you through this trauma.

Get professional help. Not only can talk therapy help you with your emotional pain, it just might help you stay alive. Research finds that group therapy for people recovering from heart surgery and heart attacks reduces death rates during the first three years of recovery, and two weekly hours of psychotherapy over seven weeks reduced the rate of rehospitalization by 60 percent.

Look for a talk therapist with experience treating survivors of heart disease. Schedule your therapy appointments for the afternoon, when you have time to reflect on the weight of the day.

If you don't have the financial ability to pay for mental health therapy, consider joining a survivor support group with others who have been through this experience. Mended Hearts (www.mendedhearts.org), a national volunteer support group for heart patients and their loved ones, is one such group. Your local chapter of the American Heart Association (1-800-AHA-USA-1) might also be able to help you find a support group near you. Other options include life coaches and religious counselors.

Use your fear as motivation to get healthy. Take the medication prescribed by your doctor. Change your diet. Exercise. Do all the steps in this book. Do what you can to reduce the likelihood of facing this challenge again.

Practice deep breathing. Breathe in through your nose and, like a baby, let your belly inflate as your lower lungs expand with the air. Then continue to fill your lungs as your rib cage and then your entire chest cavity expand, all the way up to your collarbones. Then slowly release the air. Take at least four or five breaths. This will relax and slow your pulse and lower your blood pressure. I still practice this deep breathing, even though it's years later and I'm no longer depressed. I do it whenever I feel anxious.

Learn meditation. Meditation is often taught at medical centers because it reduces the perception of physical pain, soothes anxiety, and lifts depression.[8] You can learn meditation by taking a class. See if your local hospital offers one. Many of these courses are covered by insurance. You can also purchase audiotapes online. Or you can try any one of these simple meditation exercises:

- Drink water. Slowly swallowing water throughout the day refreshes you and relaxes you, and you can picture the water filling your blood vessels and making them strong.
- Close your eyes and focus your attention on the sensation of breath as it comes in and out your nose. Feel the cool sensation as the air comes in and the warm sensation as it goes out.
- Close your eyes and count to four as you slowly inhale, and back down to zero as you exhale. You can count higher (to five, six, seven, eight, or more) as needed, depending on the natural length of your inhalation and exhalation.
- Use a two-word mantra. It can be something that means something to you, such as, "I'm well." Or it can be two sounds, such as "so hum," which means "I am that" in Sanskrit. Mentally focus on the sound of the first word as you inhale and the second word as you exhale.
- Do a body scan. Mentally go from head to toe, focusing all your attention on how various parts of your body feel, including your scalp, eyes, throat, fingertips—everything. It's like going on a tour of your body, but without any preconceived expectations. You might find that some parts of your body really hurt, are tight, or just feel uncomfortable. Try to notice those sensations without judgment. Try not to attach the sensation of discomfort to a thought, such as, "Oh no, this hurts. What is going to happen to me?" Just experience it, and then move on to the next body area. This will teach you to relax into discomfort as well as how to mentally shift your focus onto less uncomfortable parts of your body.

It doesn't matter which type of meditation you choose. What does matter is that you do it regularly. Practice every day for about ten to twenty minutes. That way you'll perfect the technique and be able to use it to calm yourself when you are feeling anxious. In lieu of meditation, you can also try self-hypnosis[9,10,11] or another relaxation technique.

Watch movies. They can take your mind off your condition, especially during the initial weeks postsurgery. Just make sure to avoid death and destruction, at least until you are feeling better. In the beginning, I could not watch any movie with violence, even though I'd loved violent dramas before my surgery. If I saw someone die on screen, I thought, "That could be me." So *The Godfather* and *The Sopranos* were out. Romantic comedies were in. Yes, I'll admit it. I watched chick flicks during my recovery! Jamie loved it. We watched *The Family Man, My Big Fat Greek Wedding,* and *The American President,* among others. It wasn't until I became more physically fit that I felt strong enough to watch violent movies again.

Listen to motivational tapes. I loved to listen to books on tape by Joan Borysenko, Deepak Chopra, and Norman Cousins. These tapes allowed me to reach into my soul and organize my thinking about surviving. Other great motivational gurus include Wayne Dyer, the Dalai Lama, and Jon Kabat-Zinn. Check the resource list in Chapter 13 for a suggested reading and listening list.

Write it down. Before I knew I was going to write a book, I somehow understood that recounting my experience would be therapeutic. I would sit down, write for a while, put it away, and then pull it back out again and read it over. I wrote about running in the park the day I experienced the chest pain that eventually led to me having a bypass. I wrote about various problems I was having at work. I mentally went back in time and wrote about the year leading up to my surgery in an effort to purge myself of some of the bottled-up stress that probably led to my heart problems. I wrote about September 11, which I'd witnessed. I wrote about all the people I interacted with in the initial weeks after my surgery. Doing this allowed me to see what I was going through in black and white, so I could more rationally analyze the events and imprint them on my mind.

Keep a pen and paper or your laptop (whatever works!) near you. Write down whatever is going through your mind once a day, especially on the days you are feeling dreadful. Quite often we hold some thoughts inside that we are too scared to voice to others, even our closest loved ones. Putting them on paper can allow us to see that we are normal. Take your journal with you when you go to see your therapist.

Take a vacation. Geographic therapy can work wonders. During my recovery, Jamie and I vacationed at her parents' home in California. It was just what I needed. It got me away from my worries. No one could visit me. I did not have to answer the phone. No one knew the old me. Jamie's father, Martin Colby, was very supportive. He and I talked daily, and I started to feel like a man again when I was with him. I could just relax and be myself. It improved my appetite, and encouraged me to exercise without the need of physical therapy, which, at that time, reminded me a bit too much of what I was coming back from.

Get a massage. Swedish massage and many other types of bodywork help you heal both physically and mentally. Research conducted in the United Kingdom determined that a fifteen-minute massage reduced both pain and anxiety in the hour posttreatment.[12,13] In a separate East Carolina University study, massage was shown to reduce blood pressure.[14] If you've just had a stent inserted, you probably do not need to take any precautions, but if you are recovering from a bypass, make sure to mention this to the therapist so the therapist knows to be very gentle, particularly around your incision.

Fill your home with the scent of lavender. When biopsy patients in a New York University Medical Center study sniffed lavender through their oxygen masks during surgery, they reported a much higher satisfaction rate with pain relief postsurgery, compared to biopsy patients who did not get lavender therapy.[15] Additional research indicates that lavender may boost self-esteem and reduce anxiety.[16,17] You can benefit from this therapy by purchasing lavender oil, placing two to four drops of it in three cups of boiling water, and then inhaling the steam. You can also add a few drops to your bathwater.

Even though it's now been years since my bout with depression, aromatherapy is still critically important to me. I still put lavender on my pillow some nights to help improve my sleep.

Find reasons to laugh. Laughter can lift your mood, distract you from your pain, and help you relax.[18] Watch funny movies. Read joke books. Ask loved ones to tell you funny stories about their lives. When I was recovering, Jamie bought me CDs and DVDs by my favorite comedian, Jackie Mason. I used to put one of his CDs in whenever I was in the car, and I would laugh until I cried, and then I would laugh even more.

Lean on your furry friends. Research shows that pets are good for us. People with dogs and cats tend to have lower blood pressure than people who don't, for example. During my recovery, Mady, our four-pound teacup Yorkshire terrier, played a huge role in lifting my spirits. Whenever

JAMIE'S ADVICE FOR CAREGIVERS

Use these tips to keep your loved one optimistic:

- Screen the greeting cards that people send. I only gave Marc the cards with uplifting messages. I nixed any card that seemed like a sympathy card.
- Rent uplifting movies. Marc has always loved action films, but I made sure the action films he watched during his recovery had the theme of someone overcoming adversity. Think Rocky. Think Rambo.
- Screen the gifts that people send your loved one. Some people sent Marc really heavy reading material, such as *The Prophet*. It's a great book, but not necessarily a great read for someone who is recovering from heart surgery.
- Don't read your spouse his horoscope. Sure, some of them are uplifting, but some just aren't.
- Give your spouse an inspiring nickname. My friend Maureen Walsh started calling Marc "Rambo." She would say, "Nothing bad can happen to you. You are Rambo. You can handle anything." It was just what he needed to hear. It still makes him feel like a superhero!

Jamie would leave the house, Mady was my constant companion. She'd never wanted to lie on my chest before, but just a day after my surgery she gently snuggled her small, warm body over my incision. It was better than any medicine. Pets seem to be intuitive, and they seem to know what we need before we know it ourselves.

Use your faith to your advantage. Many of my cancer patients have asked me whether there is any benefit to attending church or temple. Various research studies have documented a strong connection between the mind and body, a science that is known as psycho-immunology. Research also shows that people who are religious or spiritual tend to have less stress and live longer than people who are not. If you are a spiritual person, count this in your favor. Everything that you do to improve your emotional health will also help improve your physical health.

Don't be afraid to ask for medication. If natural remedies don't work, you may need an antidepressant. Years ago antidepressants were not recommended for people with heart disease because they disturbed heart rhythms and could weaken the heart. Newer antidepressants (like Prozac and Zoloft), however, are considered safe. Your doctor needs to find the one that is right for you. It will take about three to six weeks for you to notice a positive effect. You need to be patient. In my opinion, it is better to rely on a psychiatrist or psychopharmacologist for this than your primary care physician or your cardiologist. This is your brain, not your heart.

Pinpoint Your True Friends

Not long after my surgery, a colleague paid me a visit. He was a ten-year cancer survivor, and he said, "Marc, one of the most important things you must do is also the hardest. In this life there are some people who are true friends and there are others who are not. Get rid of all of the nots. Only focus on maintaining relationships with people who really support you."

It was among the best advice I ever received.

It would be nice if all our family and friends were supportive, loving, and just what we need. Unfortunately, it's just not the case. Some people are downers. Some people bring out our worst fears. Some people generate tension or anxiety. Some—usually coworkers—are looking at our every weakness, trying to uncover our faults.

I'll talk more about issues with coworkers in Chapter 9. For now, just know that people at the office are rarely your closest friends. This is especially true of the people who competed with you at work—the ones who vied for the same job titles and promotions.

They are not the people you need to surround yourself with post-surgery (or ever, really).

You need the support of people who love you, who will listen to your most irrational fears and respond *always* by telling you that you are going to recover, that you will be all right, that "we" will take care of this and get through this together. You may find that you do not have as many of these types of friends and loved ones as you may think.

Before my bypass, I took many of my everyday relationships for granted. I never stopped to think about how my coworkers felt about me. I rarely thought about my ongoing relationship with my family. Yet after my bypass I realized I no longer would have the time and energy that I once had. I had to make some careful choices about which relationships were worth continuing and which ones were not. Of course, my family was a given. I was and still am madly in love with my wife. I wanted to continue to be a good father to my children and devoted son to my mother.

But friendships and acquaintances were another story. I thought about friends and coworkers. Who was for me? Who was against me? When push came to shove, I realized that a lot of people were not there for me. During my life, they had seemed like close friends, but when I needed someone to confide in, someone to listen to my deepest fears, someone to tell me that everything would be okay, they were notably absent from my life. I realized that I did not need to put so much energy into maintaining so many relationships. In fact, the only relationships that mattered were the people who deeply loved me, the people I deeply loved, and the people who understood my need to embark on a new and unfamiliar chapter in my life: my "Chapter 2." As it turned out, only a small number of people met that description.

I consider myself lucky, because my family, especially my wife, Jamie, was there for me. I've counseled many cancer patients who did not have the same experience. Breast cancer survivors have told me that their husbands did not offer any extra help as they recovered from surgery. These survivors told me that their husbands would not touch them or look at them naked with the lights on. In their new world after surgery, these unfortunate patients realized that their spouses fell into the "against them" category. That's a very painful realization, and one I'm fortunate to not have had to deal with.

Think about the people in your life. Who is for you? Who looks out for you? Who takes up the slack? Who has your back? Who is there to listen? Concentrate all your efforts on those relationships. Accept visits from people who make you feel whole. Only allow positive people who make you feel good about yourself and your life into your circle of recovery. Unless you are very lucky, you may find that your circle of supporters is not very large.

Keep in mind that certain types of visitors can be exceptionally problematic. For instance, if your parents are still alive, you might need to develop a strategy for dealing with them that allows you to feel comfortable and allows them to know you are okay. Parents become very scared when their children—even their fifty-year-old children—become sick. Most parents cannot mask this fear and concern, and so they are not always the optimal visitors early in your recovery.

Use this advice to help build a truly supportive network of friends and loved ones.

Go online. Find discussion boards and virtual support groups for people with heart disease. In particular, check out a site called CarePages (www.carepages.com). On this site, you or your spouse can create a page about your recovery. You can write a blog about what you are going through, post photos, and even offer suggestions of what you would like people to do (send cards, call, and say, "It's so good to talk to you!" and so on) and what you would not like people to do (spend hours with you, tell you that you look "thin" or "sick," or talk about work).

Keep visits short. Ask visitors to plan to spend fifteen minutes or fewer with you, particularly in the beginning when you are feeling fatigued. If you do not feel comfortable asking visitors to leave, ask a loved one to do it for you.

Limit your visitors. Create a list of people you would like to see and people you definitely do not want to see. Then when people call and ask to visit, your spouse can look at the list and say, "Oh yes, come right over" or "He's not ready for visitors just yet. I'll be in touch when he is."

Even with a stent, you might be up and about quickly, but you still have to recover both physically and psychologically and be careful about who you surround yourself with.

Ask your spouse to prep your visitors. Most people don't intend to scare you or bring you down. They think they are being helpful but, in some cases, they are so uncomfortable that the wrong things come out of their mouths by accident. Most are just as afraid as you are—afraid that it will happen to them. So they ask you lots of details to make themselves feel better, but these are details that make *you* feel worse.

If your spouse preps them beforehand with a list of what to say and what not to say, their visits will go more smoothly.

As you figure out who your true friends really are (and you will), you may face some gray areas. There probably will be some people who mean well but who say the most annoying things. If you're not quite ready to end a relationship with one of these people, then be assertive and explain how these remarks make you feel. Below are comebacks I've used over the years for comments that are typical postsurgery.

Comment: "Stop talking about your illness. It gets to be a burden for everyone around you."

What to say: "It's important for me to talk about my illness. This is part of my recovery."

Comment: "I understand you had a heart attack" (but you didn't).

Comeback: "No, I didn't have a heart attack. I had angina, which is a medical term for chest pain. My heart muscle is still good, and now it works even better."

Comment: "You had open-heart surgery. You'll never be the same."

Comeback: "Yes, I did have surgery. At least I know what my heart looks like inside and what it's capable of. Do you?" Of all the comebacks, I used this one the most. It was most effective with my co-workers.

What should people definitely not say? Well, you don't want people to ask you what one physician friend of mine asked me about a week after my surgery: "What does it feel like to know you are going to die in the next year or two?" Thanks for the pep talk, right? I couldn't even speak after he asked me that, I was so upset. Here are some others:

- What do you think caused your heart disease? Did you have a terrible diet?
- You look really frail. Are you sure you are okay?
- Do you think you will ever be well enough to work again?
- Will you fully recover?
- Do we need to replace you?
- You seem impaired.

Only see visitors when your spouse is around. That way your spouse can usher someone out the door if needed. You might feel too guilty to tell visitors that you've had enough, but chances are your spouse can do it more easily.

❋ **BACK TO LIFE R$_x$** ❋

To boost your mood naturally:

- Walk outdoors
- Use lavender
- Snuggle with a pet
- Try meditation or deep breathing
- Watch funny movies
- Use a journal
- Sign up for talk therapy
- Try acupuncture

5

Step 3:
Get Out

AS I RECOVERED, MY HOME BECAME A SAFE ZONE. THE IDEA OF GOING outdoors filled me with anxiety.

I didn't look my best. I'd lost weight. I looked pale and tired. I did not feel as strong as I once had. When I looked in the mirror during my initial weeks after surgery, I was not fond of the Marc who stared back. I was gaunt and weak-looking. I didn't want anyone else to see the Marc I saw in the mirror.

I also feared the great outdoors. I worried about the crush of people I might encounter on the street. Would someone jostle me and, if so, would I lose my balance? Would I trip over something? Would everyone stare at me? What if I got too tired and could not make it back to my apartment?

Still, I knew I needed to get out. Doing so would be a major step in my recovery. I couldn't stay holed up in my apartment forever. I knew that sunlight, movement, fresh air, and a change in scenery were just what I needed for my mood. I knew that seasonal affective disorder was caused by lack of sunlight, as sunlight triggers the brain to produce more of the mood-boosting chemical serotonin. Exercise—even gentle exercise such as walking—has been shown to help lift depression.

I needed to get outside. As a doctor I knew I didn't have a choice.

Your First Time

Before I tell you what to do when you get out for the first time, I want to humble myself by telling you what not to do. You don't do what I did, just a week after my surgery. Jamie was out food shopping. Here I was, the chief of surgery, the marathoner, and the family stalwart. I was laid up. I was alone, and I was feeling sorry for myself. Jamie had been hinting that she'd like to take me outdoors for a walk.

I thought, "I need to make sure I'm up for this. I need to make sure I'm strong enough to go for a walk outside with my wife." I worried about possibly "failing" on the walk, of embarrassing my wife and even further destroying my self-esteem. You would have thought someone was grading me on my effort!

So I did something that—now years later—doesn't even make sense to me. I left my apartment and I walked down and then back up many flights of steps in my apartment building. I went from the twentieth floor down to the twelfth and back up.

Let me just say two words about this idea: "Bad move."

It was one of the dumbest things I've ever done. In my defense, I was still on pain meds. I wasn't thinking clearly. I wasn't in my usual state of mind.

By the time I got back to my apartment, my heart rate was 150. It would not come down. I thought, "What did I do?"

I knew the surgeon had sewn new grafts to my aorta with fine thread that is placed at precise intervals to prevent the leakage of blood. Although it's rare for these fine links to rupture seven days after surgery, I still worried that that the sudden increase in heart rate and blood pressure from my stair climbing might break the stitching, causing my grafts to come undone.

This probably would not have happened in reality, but the fear that set in over what I might have done to my heart kept my blood pressure and heart rate up for the next twenty-four hours.

I didn't leave the apartment again for two more weeks. By then Jamie was doing everything she could to get me out of the apartment short of yelling "Fire!" She finally asked me one day, "Can you help me with something?"

It was the perfect question, because it called to my sense of manhood. Of course I could help my wife with something, right? She asked me to walk with her to the corner, to help her pick out thank-you notes. I agreed, got dressed, and hid under a baseball cap. I'd lost about twenty pounds by then. I had my pants pulled up to my chest! I'd cinched my belt as tightly as it would go, but I still had to hold on to my pants to keep them from sliding down. I shuffled my feet. I felt like I was eighty years old, and apparently I looked it!

When I got to the store, I had to sit and rest as I watched my wife handle all the transactions. I felt so pathetic, but I reminded myself that at least I was outside and alive and that I had more life ahead of me.

The woman helping us said, "Your father does not look well. Is he okay?" Jamie's father? Me? It wasn't what I wanted or needed to hear. I knew she was right. I probably looked older than Jamie's father. I could not respond to her comment.

On the way back, I felt as if everyone was staring at me, wondering what this decrepit old man was doing with this young, sexy woman.

Still, I'd made it four city blocks, and that built my confidence. It inspired me to take a six-block walk the following day, with some of it uphill. From there I walked every day or every other day as long as the weather was good. With each walk, I slowly increased my distance. It was during these walks that I realized I needed a proper rehabilitation program if I was ever going to feel like my former fit self again. I knew I had to make time for it, too. Otherwise I risked becoming a cardiac cripple.

How to Get Out

To prepare for your first outdoor excursion, use this advice.

Visualize the experience. Get as calm as possible. Close your eyes and breathe deeply until you feel your heart rate slow and your muscles relax. It's very important to breathe correctly. As you take in a breath, try to bring it to the very bottom of your lungs by causing your tummy to expand. Then your rib cage will expand outward next. The very last part of your torso to fill with air should be your upper lungs, in your chest and collarbone area.

Then slowly exhale. This is the best method for decreasing blood pressure and slowing your pulse.

Once you are relaxed, imagine yourself walking outdoors. Try to use all your senses to make the experience as real as possible. What do you see, smell, feel, and hear? Does your heart speed up? What do you think when this happens? Notice how those thoughts affect your level of tension. If you start to feel tense, stop the visualization and return to deep breathing. Once you relax again, go back to the visualization. Once you can visualize an outdoor experience without getting tense, try a short outdoor excursion.

Clear things with your doctor. Find out whether you need to time your walks around your medication schedule.

Ignore the other people. Your mind will tell you that everyone you pass is staring at you. You think this because you feel so different, and so vulnerable. In reality, some people may be staring at you, particularly if they know you and wonder how you are recovering. Many people, however, probably won't notice you any more than they notice the sidewalk or grass.

Expect your first social interactions to be a challenge. About three weeks after my surgery, Jamie and I met two good friends at a restaurant. Even walking the single block to meet them was, for me, a challenge. They drove. I knew I didn't look like myself, but these were close friends. I assumed they would understand and support me. They arrived complaining about the traffic and the drive, never thinking, "Wow, how did Marc do this? That's great that he is out."

Throughout the dinner, I dealt with the following comments:

You really lost a lot of weight.

Will you ever go back to work?

How does it feel to almost die?

What was it like to have your chest cracked open?

Aren't you petrified to close your eyes at night and worried that they will never open?

The husband in this duo was a hand surgeon, colleague, and a trusted friend. If he could be so inadvertently cruel, anyone can. Arm yourself with answers because even your closest friends can seem like your worst enemies. That's why it's so important for your loved one to prep everyone, explaining what types of comments are helpful and what types are anything but.

You can't completely prevent people from asking or saying hurtful things, but you can prevent some of them. For instance, your spouse might ask the neighbors not to comment on how you look, other than to say something like, "You look great" or "It's so good to see you out and about." Depending on how you feel, you might ask your neighbors to ignore you altogether. As you walk, your spouse might further ward off comments by saying things like, "Hey, good to see you. He's doing great."

Try to anticipate questions and your responses to them. Sometimes you might feel like answering questions such as, "When will you be well again?" Sometimes you won't. If you are not in the mood to talk, just use one of these answers:

"I'm great. Thanks for asking."
"Don't worry. I'm great, thanks."

Pick a short, flat initial route. The slightest incline can seem like Mount Everest during the initial weeks after surgery or a heart attack. You want your first walk to make you feel successful and strong, so pick something you know you can do. You might walk to the mailbox and back. You might walk to the corner and back. Start with what you can mentally and physically handle, and progress from there.

Don't walk alone. Take someone with you. That way, if you start to panic, your loved one's touch and encouraging words can help bring you

I wanted to know that Marc's surgery had worked before we went out for a walk. For my personal sanity, I needed to know—without a doubt—that his coronary arteries were clear of blockages and that plenty of oxygenated blood was getting to his heart muscle.

So I scheduled a doctor's appointment before our first lengthy outing, and I asked Marc's doctor to suggest a test that would best show us that Marc's heart was indeed fixed. His doctor suggested an echocardiogram (see page 114 for a detailed description of this test), and he was able to do one right there in the office.

I'd been in the room just a few weeks earlier, when Marc had his first echocardiogram, the one that had revealed the extensive blockages that led to his bypass. Now I was in the room for his second, and boy, was it worth it. When I saw his blood flowing so freely and easily on the screen, I immediately felt a sense of peace. We could both see that his heart was pumping properly, and we both knew he would be okay.

back to reality. Let your walking partner know how you are doing, so he or she can suggest future walks that match your stamina and confidence.

Lose your iPod. You need to be alert in all your surroundings if you are going to regain your courage to go outside. You can't afford to trip or be startled by a car or bicycle. Save the iPod until you are fully recovered.

Talk to yourself. Talking yourself through your first walk outdoors is similar to talking yourself through the night. As your heart rate speeds up, you might worry, "Will I get that pain again? Will I be able to get back home without dropping dead?" If the walking feels especially difficult, you may also find yourself doubting your recovery: "If I can't even walk down the street, how am I ever going to return to work? How will I make a living? How will I support my family?"

Remind yourself that your heart is stronger and healthier than it was before. Tell yourself that you *will* come back, that you will get home. Remind yourself that your loved one is with you, that you are not alone, and that if something does happen, help is by your side. Tell yourself, "I'm out of the house. This is good. This is important. If I don't face this fear and learn how to leave the house, I will not be able to live the next chapter of my life."

How to Get Stronger and Stronger

Once you've gotten outdoors once, do it regularly. Walk a little longer each time, building up to a daily walk of at least twenty minutes. Not only is the exercise good for your heart, but walking outdoors gets you sunlight and social interaction—all of which can help boost your mood. The better your mood, the healthier your heart.

As you build up your endurance and strength, use these pointers:

- If you live in a small town or city, build up to walking to a specific location in order to accomplish a given task, such as to the bank or to a store. This will give you a sense of purpose and help you feel more in control of your life.
- In the beginning, make your outdoor excursions during the day, especially once you are alone. You will feel more in control. You'll be much

less likely to feel as if you are going to trip or become startled if you can see where you are going.

- Bring water with you. I have found that water is the elixir of life. It helps dilute your blood volume, making your blood less viscous. It also fills your vascular tree, the blood vessels that lead to and away from your heart. The less dehydrated you are, the more easily blood flows throughout your body and, most important, to your heart. This reduces the demand on your heart. Watery, fluid-filled blood is easier to pump.

- Carefully think about your routes before you tackle them. Is there a hill, even just a slight incline? Will your environment present any obstacles? For example, when you are still weak from surgery and sore from the incision, you may not want to tackle the grocery store, where you can easily become fearful of other people's carts.

How to Navigate the Grocery Store

Oh, the grocery store. It was such a mundane place before my diagnosis. Afterward? It was filled with stress.

Simple movements such as putting groceries in my cart took a lot out of me. I also lacked the mental alertness to find what I needed on the shelf. I would stand and stare at boxes and boxes and boxes of cereal, and I'd feel frustrated because I couldn't seem to find the one box that said Cheerios.

And the other shoppers with their carts! They were such careless drivers. How had I not noticed this before? It seemed as if they were all trying to ram their carts into my chest on purpose!

It would have been easy to just let Jamie do all of the shopping, but I knew I had to face the situation. I knew shopping for my own groceries was one of the best ways to take charge of my health. One of my mantras is: You are what you eat. I knew my diet was very important for maintaining my heart's health.

Here's how I got over my fear of the grocery store:

Build up to it. At first try going to the grocery store for just a couple items. It's better to go to the store once every day for a while—and feel successful and confident about the experience—than to go once a week but end up feeling tired, weak, and defeated.

Use a cart. It doesn't matter if you can hold both items in the crook of your arm. Use a cart anyway. It will both give you support and provide a protective cocoon that insulates you from the jostling of other shoppers.

Get help. Don't be afraid to ask for help, say, to reach something that's up high. Either ask another shopper or a store employee.

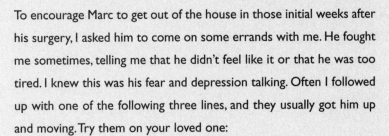

Getting Back to Yard Work

Once you feel up to it and your doctor gives you the okay, tackle outdoor activities, even lawn mowing. Many people recovering from surgery avoid mowing their lawn, but research done at Baylor Hamilton Heart and Vascular Hospital in Dallas determined that none of the bypass patients studied experienced heart rhythm problems after using a nonmotorized push mower.

Slowly work up to it, tackling it when you are ready, and in small steps. Again, talk to your doctor about it first to make sure that your wound is fully healed and that you have the clearance for mild to moderate exercise. Also, listen to your body, only doing as much as your strength allows. Use a gas-driven mower and ask someone else to start it for you (your chest may be too sore to pull the starter). You might just do a piece of your yard at first, and ask a family member or neighbor to finish the rest. Eventually, once you finish the whole yard, you'll have majorly improved your self-worth. You'll feel like a man again.

Note, however, that snow shoveling is a different story entirely. Unlike other activities, snow shoveling dramatically increases the demand on the heart. The weight of the snow on the shovel coupled with the twisting motion used to lift and toss the snow causes your heart rate and blood pressure to increase very, very quickly. It puts a tremendous stress on your heart. So many people have died from heart attacks during this activity that it's probably best to invest in a snowblower or a shoveling service.

Get Behind the Wheel of the Car

Jamie drove me to all my appointments the first six weeks post-op. That's a lot of chauffeuring around, as I had roughly five appointments every week. In the beginning, having her drive seemed to make sense. My breastbone was healing. The last thing I needed was to get into an accident and have my chest make contact with the steering wheel. Six weeks post-op, however, it was time for me to get past this fear. It was becoming irrational, and Jamie knew it.

So as we approached the car one day, she said, "You drive. I'll get in the passenger's seat." I told her, "No, you drive. I'll drive next time." I still felt insecure about getting behind the wheel. She calmly said, "Marc, you can drive. You drive."

I thought everything would have been a lot easier if she had just kept driving me around. I liked the idea of Mrs. Jamie Driving Dr. Marc a lot better than I liked the idea of trying to drive myself. She seemed to read my thoughts and said, "Marc, you're ready." That was what I needed to hear.

So I got behind the wheel. As I pulled onto the street, I thought, "Am I seeing clearly? What if something happens? Can I make it to where I need to go without a health problem, and what if I can't?" I was hypervigilant, driving exactly the speed limit and worrying about every single traffic law. You would have thought I was a sixteen-year-old who'd just gotten his license.

It's normal to feel insecure about certain tasks that you could easily do before your cardiac event. To get past that insecurity, you need to convince yourself that you can drive—and you really can. Cardiac disorders only slightly increase your driving risk, assuming you've been treated.[1,2,3] This increase is so slight that University of Toronto researchers have used these results to prove that bus drivers can safely return to work after having a heart attack.[4]

You need to get over your fear of the car. Without doing so, you'll end up becoming a shut-in, especially if you live in the suburbs. Isolation is not good for your heart. It's probably a good idea to refrain from driving for one week after angioplasty and one month after a heart attack or bypass surgery, and six months after having a pacemaker inserted.[5] How do you know whether or not you are ready? If you've had no chest pain or irregular heart rhythms for four weeks and your doctor keeps wondering why your spouse continually accompanies you to your appointments, you are ready.

The thing is, you really need to believe this, and the only way to make that happen is to tell yourself this sort of thing over and over again. As I drove, I repeatedly said to myself, "I am up and around. I am well. I can

LIFE PRESERVER

Studies show that the people who are most likely to have heart attacks tend to commute to work by car, compared to people who walk, bike, or take public transportation to work. Why? For one thing, people who walk or bike to work are getting more exercise, and exercise is good for your heart. Second, commuting—especially in traffic—can be anger-producing, and anger is bad for your heart. Third, the smog produced by traffic is just as bad for your heart as cigarette smoke. A German study of nearly seven hundred people determined that the more time men spent in a car the more likely they were to have a heart attack, with a high percentage of men suffering heart attacks within an hour of being exposed to traffic!

How do you reduce your dependence on the car? Try any or all of the following:

- Investigate public transportation. Many cities offer free bus service during smog alerts. Keep in mind that public transportation will make you feel somewhat vulnerable—especially early in your re-covery— if crowds of people are involved.
- Walk or ride a bike for short trips.
- Carpool.
- Consider moving closer to work or working closer to your home.
- Patronize stores and services that are closer to your home or work.

see and walk and talk. I am well." I kept telling myself over and over again that I was okay, that I was normal, and that I knew how to drive a car.

Start with a very short trip. You can even just drive around the block. Drive on relatively quiet roads first, too. Like you did when you took driver's education, start with easy routes and slowly work your way up to highway driving and finally rush-hour traffic.

Once you get used to being behind the wheel, be careful of overconfidence. About four months post-op, I drove Jamie to the Hamptons in Long Island, a three-hour drive from New York City, where we live. We had a new car, and I took it out on the highway for the first time. It was a beautiful day. I opened the car up and was driving 110 or 120 miles per hour. I felt so alive, until a police officer pulled me over and wrote me a speeding ticket. As he threatened to revoke my license if I ever got caught going that fast again, I tried to explain why I had done it, that it was an aberration. "Let me explain what happened to me," I told the officer. "I just needed to know that I was alive." He wasn't interested. He gave me a citation.

Travel by Plane

Traveling by plane presents a unique set of problems. Not only must you navigate the airport and transport heavy bags, you also may battle the fear of flying. I, for one, worried about the lack of oxygen in the pressurized cabin. I wondered, "Will my red blood cells have enough oxygen to nourish my heart muscle?" I also knew that some people—even people without heart disease—develop clots in their legs during flying, clots that can travel to the lungs, heart, or brain.

Use this advice:

- Again, visualize the trip ahead of time. Try to take in every possible detail. See yourself at the airport, boarding the plane, and sitting down. Whenever you feel anxious during the visualization, return to deep breathing until you calm down. Then continue with the visualization.
- Continually remind yourself of the reason for your trip. You might simply say, "This is good for me. I need to do this. I am going somewhere where I will be safe and protected. I will be there soon."
- Ask for assistance at the airport, especially during your initial trips. It's

part of your recovery. You can use motorized transportation to the gate, if needed, and even get help with your bags.

- If the flight is a long one, consider talking to your doctor about anti-anxiety medication or a sleeping pill to help you get through the trip. Also, be sure to walk up and down the aisle during the flight and take an aspirin to prevent blood clots in your legs (a common problem during a long flight, even in people without heart disease).

No matter what type of obstacle you face outdoors, remember this: Take baby steps. Start small, tackling one challenge at a time. Every time you take a small step in the right direction, celebrate that success. Use that positive reinforcement—along with the positive reinforcement you receive from your loved ones and physician—to remind yourself that you really can get stronger and healthier—and that soon you will be fully recovered.

❋   BACK TO LIFE R$_x$ ❋

- Get outdoors as soon as possible.
- Choose a short, flat route.
- Take someone with you.
- Go during the day.
- Think positively: "I can do this. I'll make it."
- Go a little farther each time.
- Celebrate each baby step.

6

Step 4:
Survive Doctors'
Appointments

HEART DISEASE RUNS IN MY FAMILY. MY FATHER AND PATERNAL grandfather both died of heart attacks. My maternal grandfather and grandmother and my mother all had heart disease, with my grandfather surviving several heart attacks. As a result, long before I had any symptoms, I visited any number of cardiologists for testing.

I got regular blood draws. I got stress tests. I did heart scans and calcium scoring. Because I was a physician, I knew what tests were available. I knew how to ask for them. I was my own best advocate.

Yes, the marathoning gave me a false sense of invincibility. (*If I can do this, there's no way anything could possibly be wrong with my heart!*) At the same time, I underwent test after test after test because I needed to know for sure. I didn't want any doubt in my mind. I needed to know that I was healthy.

Because academic medicine can keep you on the move, I changed jobs often and lived in many different parts of the country. I ended up undergoing testing from many different doctors, including Arthur Agatston, M.D., who later wrote *The South Beach Diet*. More than twenty-two years before my bypass surgery, when I was still in my thirties, it was Dr. Agatston who did a heart scan and determined that I had more than a normal amount of plaque on my coronaries for a man my age. It was a wake-up call, and it got me to overhaul my diet and learn how to relax. I trusted Dr. Agatston and knew I had to pay attention.

My relationships with these cardiologists were a little different than most patients' relationships with their doctors, though. I did more than participate in my care. At times I treated myself—because I could.

For instance, I was diagnosed with high blood pressure in my early forties. I was taking medication for it and I monitored my pressure at home. Whenever my pressure went up, I altered my medication dosage and got it back down.

I also started aspirin therapy when I read that it could prevent heart attacks and stroke. I once even prescribed a cholesterol-lowering medicine to myself. I always discussed these matters with my cardiologist. I kept nothing secret, but I was definitely serving, in part, as my own doctor.

It wasn't until my bypass that I truly knew what it felt like to be a patient, to completely give up all sense of control and trust my health and well-being to another person. In the days leading up to my bypass and afterward, I felt myself losing power. I was weak, humbled, and depressed.

I didn't like not being in control. I didn't like it at all.

But I had no choice.

The Doctor Becomes a Patient

During my first office visit after the surgery, my physician checked my wound and prescribed beta-blockers to slow my heart. He adjusted my blood pressure medicine, too.

Unlike in the years before, when I'd self-medicated, I now felt I was at my doctor's mercy. I felt like I had to listen to and do everything he suggested. If I didn't, I worried I would die.

That depressed the hell out of me, as you might imagine.

During one visit, I told my doctor that I needed to gain control of my life again. As I said it, I started to cry. Yes, me. Crying. That had never happened before, especially in front of another doctor!

He referred me to a psychiatrist, who prescribed antidepressants. That helped.

Still, each doctor's visit filled me with fear. Every single time I worried that my doctor would find something wrong. My cholesterol or blood pressure would be too high. Maybe I would fail a stress test. Maybe some scan would detect new blockages.

I eventually realized that I just had to go, and that the more often I got myself through the experience, the easier each experience would become.

You need to do the same. You absolutely need to step foot in the doctor's office and get test results—many times over—not only so you can recover physically, but also so you can recover *emotionally*. It's that clean bill of health—the healthy cardiogram or stress test results—that will provide you with the courage you need to get on with your life.

At the same time, your doctor's office may hold some bad memories. It might be the place where you first learned that you had heart problems, for instance. Also, the thought of getting a bad test result can fill you with fear. Indeed, every cell in your body may tell you, "Don't go!"

You can ease the stress of these appointments. In this chapter, I'll show you how.

The Phone: Your Lifeline

If you underwent a bypass, your cardiologist probably will schedule a checkup about six to eight weeks after your surgery to determine how well you are healing. Don't hesitate to call or schedule a visit sooner if needed. For instance, I called my doctor the day after I tried that crazy stair-climbing workout just a week after my surgery (see Chapter 5).

I called when I thought my heart was beating too quickly, whenever I felt as if my heart was skipping beats, or when I just felt that I was on an emotional roller coaster. I called when my appetite did not return, when I was relying too heavily on painkillers, when I thought I was crying too much, and even when I feared walking outdoors or talking on the phone.

These are not unusual postoperative problems, by the way, and sometimes you just need to hear that what you are going through is very normal and very treatable. You might need an adjustment in medication, an office visit so your doctor can show you just how healthy and normal you really are, or a referral to a therapist or specialist.

See or call your doctor as frequently as you need to feel comfortable with your recovery. Ask your cardiologist and cardiac surgeon for all their contact information. Find out the best way to contact them during the day and during non-office hours. Ask if your doctor checks e-mail often. If so, get his or her address, both the home and the office address. Find out the names and numbers for related office staff (such as nurse practitioners or physician's assistants) who might be able to help with your questions and concerns when your cardiologist is unavailable.

I encourage you to call your doctor whenever:

• You are worried that something is not "normal." Perhaps your heart is beating faster than usual. Perhaps you just don't feel right. Maybe your spouse thinks you are taking too much pain medication (see Chapter 4). It could be any number of nagging worries. Let your doctor ease your mind.

• You are not sure whether or not it's safe for you to do something. Is it safe to have sex? (More on this in Chapter 7.) Are you ready to drive alone? Can you exercise? Ask your doctor.

• Your wound does not seem to be healing. For instance, you might notice redness, pain, or tenderness around the wound edges.

• You have any type of overwhelming anxiety for any reason.

- Your chest hurts.
- You are worried you might be having a heart attack.
- You have fever or chills. This is not normal after heart surgery and should be addressed.
- Your heart is beating irregularly.
- You feel out of breath too often and with easy exertion.
- You have severe headaches that occur more frequently than before your procedure.

Whenever you call the office, the first words out of your mouth—before the live human being says a single thing—should be "Please do not put me on hold." Your physician's office probably put you on hold more times than you can remember before your event. Other than being annoying, however, being put on hold might not have affected you all that much. Now things are very different. Now being on hold to talk to a nurse or office personnel might be torture. It was for me. I would have a question, one that I thought was important. I called because I was already anxious to begin with, and the person on the other line couldn't even wait for me to say my name?!

Your First Checkup

You should see your cardiac surgeon the first week after surgery to check your wound. You'll see your cardiologist a few weeks later, and then at least once every few months during the first year.

During that first appointment with your cardiologist, your doctor will give you instructions on driving, returning to work, and pain medications. Also, there may be some changes in your heart medication that will become more obvious to your cardiologist after the surgery. You'll also get a

It takes a lot of courage to face doctor's appointments, especially the first one. Try making a special outing out of it. Perhaps you go can out to lunch afterward or buy something special, like a new outfit. Do something that reminds you that you still have a life to live, and a future.

schedule regarding how often to see your doctor for regular follow-ups and testing.

Your doctor is ready and waiting for you to ask questions, particularly at this initial appointment. The problem? You might have hundreds of questions, but the anxiety of seeing your doctor may cause your mind to go blank. Worse, you might focus so much on wanting to hear good news or on not wanting to hear bad news that you miss most of what your doctor has to say.

To get over the stress of appointments, use this advice:

Write down your questions ahead of time. That way, if you forget what you want to know, you can always look at your notes to jog your memory. Good questions to ask your doctor include:

- Is my heart beating well?
- Is my heart stronger than it used to be?
- Is my wound healing properly?
- Am I getting better?
- Is there anything else I should be doing for my health?
- How should I be eating? Is my diet healthful enough?
- Is it safe for me to (have sex, drive a car alone, take a trip on an airplane, etc.)?

- Is it normal for me to feel (sad, lack of appetite, listless, tired, etc.)?
- When can I exercise and what types of exercise can I do?
- How much exertion is safe?
- Can I carry a briefcase, groceries, my pet, or my grandchild?

Call ahead. Explain that you are feeling anxious and ask not to be left in the waiting room when you arrive. The longer you must wait, the worse your anxiety will become. Or ask a loved one to make the call. He or she might say something like, "My loved one is really in a funk. He might get really anxious if he has to sit around the waiting room for a long time. Is there any way we can be seen immediately?"

Schedule your appointment for the first thing in the morning. I recommend early-morning appointments for two reasons. First, you'll wait for a shorter period of time. Second, you'll get the news out of the way so you can enjoy the rest of your day. Try to schedule the appointment for before or after rush hour, however, so you avoid stress as you get to the appointment. If you can't get the first appointment in the morning, try for the first in the afternoon. Usually the office gets back on track during the lunch break, so you're less likely to wait as long for the first afternoon appointment as you would later in the afternoon.

Take a notebook with you. Write down any specific instructions your doctor offers, even if you think you can remember them later. Ask your doctor for any handouts he or she may have regarding this information. Ask your doctor to write down any complicated information—such as medication dosages and schedules—for you, so there is no confusion later on. Don't be afraid to ask your doctor to spell words that seem unfamiliar to you.

Take your iPod. If you do—despite your request—get stuck in the waiting room or in the exam room for a long period of time, put on headphones, play your favorite soothing music, close your eyes, and try to relax. Similarly, you can bring along other distractions, such as a crossword puzzle, a book, or a game.

Bring a friend or loved one. Nothing feels as scary when you have a companion sitting next to you. Have someone there with you—especially for your first major appointment—to remind you that you are okay. A spouse, best friend, or long-term romantic love interest is optimal. In lieu of a spouse, you can also turn to grown children. Just keep in mind that children can have a difficult time contemplating the frailties of a parent. They look at us parents as all-powerful people. Sitting with you in a physician's office may be even more stressful for them than it is for you.

In addition to serving as a source of emotional support for you, your loved one can:

- Bring up topics and issues with your doctor that you might be too flustered or nervous to talk about yourself. Ask a loved one to help you describe your problems (such as pain or insomnia) and get medicines that are appropriate.
- Write down what the doctor says, as you may be nervous and unable to remember it or pay attention. Ask your loved one to take notes and read them back to you later.

Wear comfortable clothing. That way it will be easy to get undressed and dressed again at the office. Wear slip-on shoes until you are comfortable enough to bend over.

Talk yourself through it. Whenever you feel anxious, remind yourself that you are making progress. It might help to go to the appointment with a prepared list of milestones. Can you walk around the block without feeling winded? Are you sleeping comfortably through the night? Are you able to get up in the morning without fear? Is your pulse regular? Does your spouse gush about the strength of the sound of your heartbeat or about the new color in your cheeks?

If you are in cardiac rehab, remind yourself how much your heart can handle. After all, exercise is the greatest stress test there is. If you can continually push yourself physically, then you already know what the tests will find—that you are healthy. This is one of the hidden benefits of cardiac rehab. Not only does it get you stronger physically, it helps you recover emotionally, too, by showing you that you are indeed healthy enough to handle life, love, and the pursuit of happiness again.

Come up with a positive mantra for yourself, one that you continually tell yourself over and over as needed. It might be any of the following:

- "I'm doing great. My doctor is just going to tell me what I already know."
- "I feel strong. I am strong."
- "I am making progress. My test results will show that."

Expect that your heart rate will rise with your doctor's every word and touch. If you feel your heart rate speeding up, remember that mantra and breathe deeply. It's okay to tell the doctor or nurse that you need a moment to pull yourself together. You will not be the first patient who has ever done so! If you feel your heart rate speeding up, focus on the sensation of breathing, on the coolness that you feel on the edge of your nostrils as you inhale. Breathe deeply five times, filling your abdomen and then your chest with air before slowly exhaling.

JAMIE'S ADVICE FOR CAREGIVERS

When taking your loved one to that initial appointment, you can do a number of things to make the whole experience go more smoothly for you both.

- Drop your loved one off at the door and ask him or her to wait as you park the car.

- Call ahead—if you've never been to this office before—and find out where the elevator is. That way you won't have to wander around looking for it. Not only can the simple problem of finding the elevator be stressful on your loved one, the act of walking longer than needed can be very fatiguing soon after surgery.

- If you think your loved one is taking too much pain medicine (see Chapter 4), call ahead and mention it to the doctor. This allows the doctor to ask the right questions and prevents you and your spouse from getting into an argument in front of the doctor.

- Continually remind your loved one that everything is going to be okay. Hold your loved one's hand. If you notice him or her getting upset, say something like, "You look so vibrant today. I can't wait to hear your doctor tell you how healthy you are."

- Speak to the doctor in private. Ask him or her to make at least one positive comment about your loved one's recovery during every visit. Doctors often get so caught up in finding and explaining what's wrong that they forget to point out what's right.

- Make a lunch date. I always booked an early lunch reservation at a nice restaurant before the lunch rush so Marc would have something pleasant to look forward to after the appointment.

When all else fails, take a sedative. Talk to your doctor about getting a prescription for Xanax or another prescription tranquilizer that will help you settle your nerves before doctor's appointments.

Understand Your Disease

Part of what's scary about heart disease is this: It's so complicated. The fear of something going wrong is a lot greater when you don't understand what's going right or wrong. It's also much more frustrating to listen to your doctor if you don't understand half the words coming out of his or her mouth. That's why I've included this primer here, so you can understand what your heart does and how.

A muscle the size of your fist, your heart works 24-7 to circulate blood throughout your body. It contains four chambers, all of which are separated by valves. The chambers on the right side of the heart take blood from the body and send it to the lungs, where cells drop off carbon dioxide and pick up oxygen. Then this newly oxygenated blood flows through the left side of the heart, which pumps it onward to the rest of your body.

The arteries that carry blood to your heart (known as coronary arteries) are very small. They can become even narrower if fatty gunk (called plaque) builds up inside them. The more these arteries narrow, the less blood can get through. When your heart doesn't get enough blood to meet its needs, it starts to hurt, and this pain is called angina. If blood flow is cut off for an extended period of time, cells in the heart start to die. This is known as a heart attack, or a myocardial infarction.

Understand Your Test Results

Get the tests you need to prove to yourself and your loved ones that you are healthy. It's important that your loved ones are as convinced of your good health as you are. Research completed at the University of Kentucky and University of California at San Francisco has found that healthy spouses who feel anxious and depressed can cause their recovering patient partners to feel just as distressed, which delays patient recovery! So get these tests as often as you need them, so you and your loved ones all feel ready to move on.

Your doctor will give you a schedule for follow-up testing, but you can get tests more often than the schedule dictates. You might want more frequent testing if:

- You are worried about your health. The tests will help ease your mind.
- You are having panic attacks and confusing them with heart attacks. Again, the tests will ease your mind, allowing you to know that it's all in your mind.

In the following pages, you'll find a rundown of the common types of tests you may need. Be an active participant in your care. Ask questions. Find out from your doctor what each test means. Look over your test results with your doctor, so you can see for yourself why your doctor thinks you are so healthy. Ask for copies of results, so you can review them at home, if needed, to build your confidence.

Stress test. This is the treadmill or stationary bike test. You should have one done within the first six months after surgery, and then at least once a year after that. Walking on the treadmill or pedaling a bike makes your heart beat faster than usual, making it easier for heart problems to be detected. As you walk or cycle, your doctor will monitor your blood pressure and heart rhythm with an EKG. (If you are too weak to exercise, your doctor can speed up your heart rate with medication.) Note that the stress test is not perfect. I had one every six months, and except for the one I had just days before my bypass, they all told me that I was healthy as a horse!

I recommend that you undergo a special type of stress test called a thallium stress test about six months after surgery. During this test, thallium—a radioactive substance—is injected into your bloodstream. Then you lie on a table under a special camera that sees the thallium and takes pictures of your heart and surrounding blood vessels. The thallium allows your doctor to see where blood is flowing and where it is not flowing. If a part of your heart is not getting enough blood, the thallium won't get to that part of the heart—and it won't show up in the picture.

Echocardiogram. During your initial postsurgery visits, you'll undergo this test to make sure that your heart is beating regularly and rhythmically and that all of the chambers are working normally. This test uses sound waves to create a moving picture that shows blood flowing through the chambers and valves of your heart. It helps your doctor see how well your heart pumps and how well the chambers and valves are working. This may be done in conjunction with a stress test.

Electrocardiogram. An EKG detects the electrical activity of the heart. It shows how fast the heart is beating, whether the heart's rhythm is normal, and whether the electrical activity is traveling through the heart normally. This may be done in conjunction with a stress test. You should have at least one EKG postsurgery. Ask your cardiologist how often you should undergo this testing afterward based on the severity of your preoperative heart status.

X-ray. You need at least one postsurgery so your doctor can make sure your heart and lungs are healthy. An X-ray can detect whether fluid is collecting around your lungs, as it did for former President Bill Clinton after his heart surgery, causing a lung to collapse.

Blood work. You should have a full blood panel done during the first few months. Go over your results with your doctor, making sure you understand your total cholesterol, LDL (bad) cholesterol, HDL (good) cholesterol, C-reactive protein (a measure of inflammation; high levels of inflammation are bad for your heart), homocysteine (elevated levels raise risk of heart disease). Here's a quick primer on all these blood markers.

If levels of any of these blood markers are elevated, your doctor might prescribe cholesterol-lowering or statin (anti-inflammatory) medication.

Total cholesterol: This is your HDL and LDL added together. For optimal health, this number should be less than 200 mg/dL.

LDL: Low-density lipoprotein or "bad" cholesterol, LDLs are transportation vehicles that carry extra cholesterol and fats in your blood. LDLs do not tend to be very careful drivers, though, and they can be somewhat lazy. They often come to rest on the lining of your arteries and get stuck, allowing debris to build up and harden into plaque. This number should be less than 120 mg/dL, although less than 100 mg/dL is ideal.

HDL: High-density lipoprotein or "good" cholesterol, HDLs carry cholesterol and fat away from your arteries and to your liver to be processed. They tend to be careful and efficient drivers. They don't tend to build up on the sides of your arteries, which is why they are called the good guys. This number should be more than 60 mg/dL.

Triglycerides: This is a type of fat that floats around in your bloodstream. Your body converts sugary foods, saturated fats, and starches into these fats. If your cells don't use them for energy, they will eventually be stored as fat, assuming they don't get stuck inside your arteries first. This number should be less than 150 mg/dL.

C-reactive protein: Your liver makes this protein in response to infection, injury, and inflammation. Of those three, inflammation raises your risk of heart disease. Assuming you are not injured or sick, a high CRP test result means one thing: there's too much inflammation in your body. The lower your CRP, the better. A healthy reading is 1 milligram per liter (mg/L). Anything between 1 and 3 is considered an intermediate risk, and anything higher than 3 puts you in the high-risk range. CRP is not as helpful after your diagnosis as it was before, because a high reading does not usually change your treatment (as you are probably already taking the medications necessary to lower CRP levels). It's also not generally a part of a standard blood panel. You may need to request that your doctor include it.

Homocysteine: This is an amino acid that, in high amounts, can irritate the lining of your blood vessels, leading to heart disease. This is not as sensitive as C-reactive protein.

Blood glucose: Your cells use glucose to make energy. When you eat a diet rich in starch, sugar, or calories, more glucose enters your bloodstream than your cells can use at any given time. Your body will convert the excess into fat and store it in your fat cells, but chronically elevated glucose can eventually lead to diabetes, which in turn raises your risk of heart disease.

Blood pressure. Your blood pressure is the force of blood against the walls of your arteries. If your arteries are narrowed as a result of plaque buildup, your blood pressure will go up due to a law of physics that you might have learned about in high school or college. It's called Bernoulli's Principle. Fluid flows faster and with greater force when it is confined to a narrow space. Think about a river. A very wide river flows slowly and smoothly. A narrow one tends to flow quickly and have a lot of rapids. It's the same with your blood vessels.

The more pressure there is inside them, the more the flow of the blood can damage the lining of your arteries, leading to even more scarring and buildup as the body attempts to repair that damage. It's a vicious cycle! High blood pressure can also cause plaque to break loose and form a deadly blood clot, which can travel to your brain (causing a stroke), your heart (causing a heart attack), or your kidneys (causing kidney failure).

Your doctor will check your blood pressure every visit. Normal blood pressure is less than 120/80 mmHg. High is anything higher than 140/90. Anything between those two is considered prehypertension. (*Hypertension* is a fancy word for high blood pressure.) If your blood pressure is elevated, your doctor might prescribe medication to bring it back down. You might find it helpful to purchase a home blood pressure monitor or frequently use one that might be available at your local drugstore or grocery store, especially if psychological stress seems to be raising your pressure. Talk to your doctor about whether such a device is worth the investment.

Body weight. Excess body fat raises your risk for heart disease in many different ways. The heavier you are, the harder it is for your heart to pump blood throughout your body, which leads to increased blood pressure. Excess body weight also makes cells less receptive to absorbing and burning blood glucose for energy, which leads to diabetes. It raises cholesterol and triglyceride levels, too. See Chapter 8 for a heart-healthy eating plan that will help you lose weight, too.

It's easy to mistake the symptoms of panic for the symptoms of heart trouble. After all, many of the symptoms can be exactly the same: chest tightness, numbness, and tingling throughout the body. Here are some ways to tell the difference:

It's probably a panic attack if . . .

- You are hyperventilating. This doesn't usually happen with a heart attack, unless, of course, you are panicking because you think you are having a heart attack.
- The pain is centered right over your heart and comes and goes, usually intensifying with breathing.
- Deep breathing gets your breathing rate and heart rate under control within five minutes. Heart attack symptoms generally persist.

It's probably a heart attack if . . .

- The chest pain feels heavy, as if a linebacker were sitting on your chest.
- The pain radiates to your chin and/or down your left arm.
- The pain lasts longer than ten minutes, or it eases only to return a few minutes later.

Nuclear heart scanning. Your physician will inject a radioactive tracer and special camera into your bloodstream. This allows your doctor to see the flow of blood through your heart and arteries. This may be done in conjunction with a stress test. Though it's not necessary, this is a good test to undergo about a year postsurgery, to make sure your heart is beating adequately and getting enough blood flow.

Angiogram. If your doctor recommends this test, dye will be injected into your bloodstream. The dye will help your arteries better show up on an X-ray, so your doctor can see if your vessels are free of blockages.

About Cardiac Rehabilitation

From the very beginning, I knew I wanted to run again. So from the very beginning, my cardiac rehabilitation program focused not just on getting me fit enough for everyday activities, but also on getting me fit enough for marathon training.

When I got back on a treadmill for the first time about three weeks after surgery, my muscles still ached and my chest still hurt. I didn't think I would be able to get back to where I once was. "Maybe I can't run another marathon again," I told myself. "Maybe my only goal should be to return to the world of running. If I can just become a runner again, that will be enough." My pulse shot from 80 beats per minute to 130 beats per minute. It had nothing to do with the physical work; the treadmill was barely in motion. The racing heartbeat stemmed from my fearful thoughts: *My God, I'm not sure I can do this. Maybe my heart is not fixed.* My cardiac therapist encouraged me to take deep breaths, which calmed me down.

This helped. I progressed to running in a rehabilitation pool, submerged in water, putting one foot in front of the other. Slowly I progressed. I advanced to running up and down steps. I started weight training, too.

And within a period of months, I was running again.

You might have no aspirations to run, but that doesn't mean you should forgo rehab. Some hospitals, cardiologists, and cardiac surgeons automatically funnel you into a cardiac rehabilitation program and some don't. If yours does not, seek out a rehab program, with plans to start rehab as soon as your doctor recommends. It will make a huge difference not only in your physical recovery, but also your emotional recovery.

Why? You don't want to live the rest of your life in fear of your heart beating quickly. There will be times when you will need to run through an airport to catch a plane, lift heavy objects (perhaps your own children), and climb up stairs. And exercise is important for your heart health. Even if you were a couch potato before your diagnosis, you cannot afford to be one now. You need to get and stay fit, and cardiac rehabilitation is the first step toward that goal.

When UK researchers followed the health outcomes of 179 patients for five years after having a heart attack, those who underwent cardiac rehab had improved their fitness. Those who did not undergo cardiac rehab, however, deteriorated and lost even more fitness.[1] A separate Japanese study determined that patients who underwent cardiac rehab had healthier cholesterol levels and less anxiety than their counterparts who did not choose this therapy.[2]

Most rehab programs allow you to work one-on-one with a physical therapist, at least in the beginning. You'll go anywhere from every day to a few times a week. You'll start with gentle stretches, to help increase your range of motion. Your therapist might also massage your chest to help increase circulation and loosen up and flatten the scar from your surgery. You'll go home with a printout of these stretches so you can do them at home.

Then you'll advance to improving your cardiovascular fitness. You might do this on a treadmill or while partially submerged in a pool. A therapist or a nurse will be with you as you exercise, monitoring your heart rate throughout. You might only last a minute or two in the beginning. Eventually you'll be able to exercise for twenty minutes or longer. Eventually you'll start a strength-training program, too.

A standard program lasts anywhere from one to three months. That's about all your insurance plan will allow. If you can afford it, I encourage you to stay in the program longer. I did mine for thirteen months. By the end of your time in cardiac therapy, you should feel as if you've developed total body fitness, so you have the confidence you need to continually build your fitness on your own.

Although you may still feel emotionally and physically drained when you start your rehab program, it's worth it. It builds the confidence you need to get on with living the rest of your life. Your therapist probably will have a better idea about what you are capable of than you will. After all, he or she has helped hundreds, if not thousands, of people just like you. This gentle encouragement will help you push yourself.

Your therapist's presence will also help you calm down when you do find yourself in a panic, as I did that first time on the treadmill. I highly recommend it. It is also your first step toward getting back into shape and starting a formal exercise program. Your family doctor or cardiologist can give you information about programs in your local area (cardiac rehabilitation is covered by most insurance companies) or you may go to the American Association of Cardiovascular and Pulmonary Rehabilitation website (www.aacvpr.org) to search for a program.

Find a rehabilitation therapist who "gets" you. Your therapist should:

- Understand you as a person and relate to you. For instance, my rehabilitation therapist had played sports and suffered numerous injuries.

He understood my mentality about wanting to run again, particularly a marathon.

- Seem confident about your recovery, so you can feel confident, too.
- Have worked with many patients with heart disease.

If you do not feel comfortable with your therapist, ask for a new one. Your recovery depends on it.

Use this advice for cardiac rehab:

Start slowly. Recognize that eventually you will not need your therapist. Now, however, it's a slow, baby-step-forward process.

Stay in rehab for at least three months. Go about two to three times a week, starting therapy long before you plan to return to work.

Make sure you can time your visits around your work schedule. Investigate early morning, lunch hour, or early evening appointments.

When to Find a New Doctor

One visit to the eye doctor many years ago taught me a lot about how patients must feel when their doctors cannot give them the information they need as quickly as possible and with as much compassion as possible. My eye exam was two years overdue, which is par for the course. Although I did a great job monitoring my heart health, I didn't do so great a job with the rest of my body. Doctors tend to do a terrible job of taking care of themselves unless they are ravaged with illness. We focus on caring for others instead.

Anyway, when my doctor dilated and examined my eyes, he calmly stated that he saw a black lesion in the back of my eye. He thought it might be a melanoma (a very deadly form of cancer). He held my hand and with a very even, tranquil tone of voice said, "We're going to get through this. I will send you to a specialist and I will be there as the specialist examines you. We will find out whether this is cancer or something else. Even if it is cancer, we're going to get through this."

I knew melanoma was deadly. I knew I could possibly lose my eyesight, something that would end my career. But he had this slight grin on his face the entire time. It was as if he knew something that I did not. It gave me a sense of inner peace.

As it turned out, the spot was not melanoma but, in fact, a harmless mole. Had that doctor not been so kind and compassionate, I probably would have not been able to remain calm throughout the experience.

Not all physicians have perfect bedside manner. They are not all as compassionate as mine was. They don't all explain complex medical information in a way the average person can understand. But that doesn't mean that you need to put up with a less than perfect doctor. You don't have to stay with a doctor you do not like.

The cardiologist who diagnosed and treated you initially may not be the doctor you stick with long term. You may have found this initial doctor in a hurry. He or she may have been the only doctor available when you were wheeled into the ER with chest pain. Now that you've had surgery, medication, and treatment, you have time to find a new cardiologist if needed.

When should you look for a new doctor? When you don't feel comfortable. Your cardiologist should not:

- Make you feel rushed
- Make you feel stupid

- Make you feel uncomfortable
- Have unfriendly office staff
- Downplay your concerns or questions or refuse to devote the time that you need

You want a doctor who:

- Makes you feel at ease
- Makes you feel welcome to ask questions
- "Gets" you
- Is willing to give you phone and e-mail information so you can reach him or her personally after hours
- Reassures you

Good doctors don't behave as if they are great. They don't try to sound or act important. Rather, good doctors make you feel completely comfortable, as if you are both on equal footing.

How do you find a new doctor? Get referrals from friends, family, your primary care physician, and, most important, other survivors. Ask other survivors, "Do you have a doctor who makes you feel comfortable?" Go online to research cardiologists in your area. Check to see if other patients have reviewed them. Contact the American Heart Association (www.americanheart.org) for a list of board-certified cardiologists near you.

Interview potential candidates. Ideally, you want a doctor who:

- May have been through this. Perhaps he or she has had a heart attack or bypass surgery. This is rare, but it can really be helpful.

- Has friendly office staff. If you have an "I don't like being here" sensation while in the waiting room or while dealing with any of the office staff, then it's probably not the right practice for you.

Remember: This is your health, your heart, and your peace of mind. You deserve to have a compassionate doctor. Don't settle for anything less.

❖ THE UNBEATABLES ❖

Chase Carter died for the first time at age twenty-nine. His heart just stopped beating and, in the middle of the dance floor at an Air Force holiday party, he fell over. Doctors managed to bring him back, but then he died again. And again. And he came back again and again. Eventually doctors determined that an electrical problem with his heart caused him to have an irregular heartbeat. They didn't provide much hope for the condition. They implanted an experimental pacemaker and told him to get his affairs in order. He probably had a year to live, tops. That was twenty-nine years ago.

When I first died at age twenty-nine, I was in denial. I was so very young. I felt invincible. I knew I might die again, but it didn't occur to me that I might die and not come back.

Then one day, I was looking at a house. My real estate agent told me she had indigestion and asked if I could drive her to a hospital. As we walked to her car, she dropped to the ground. I got her to the hospital as soon as I could, but she was already dead. She'd had a heart attack. That was a wake-up call for me.

Two weeks later, I had a nervous breakdown. I grieved the loss of my health. I asked, "Why me?" a lot, and I became very afraid. I was afraid to go to the grocery store. I was afraid to drive my car. I was afraid to walk outside. No matter what I did or where I was—whether it was at the mall or at the movies or on a date— I wondered, "What would happen if I dropped dead right here like she did?"

I wasn't so much scared of dying as I was scared of inconveniencing others. I didn't want to be in my car, cause an accident, and hurt someone else. I didn't want to be in the middle of the grocery store and cause a big ruckus.

After a while, though, I realized that I had to live my life the best way I could. For me that meant becoming a mental health counselor, teaching classes on death and dying at the local university, and then writing music. The music, called the Chase Carter Method, was based on the music and sounds I heard when I was dead and in the tunnel. That was the most beautiful music I had ever heard. It was so restful and peaceful. Other people who have crossed over also say they've heard music and wonder whether it's the sounds of angels' wings. I like to think of it as the sounds of the universe. Whatever the origin of those sounds, they are beautiful, and I try to emulate them in my music.

I've realized that in the tunnel when I am dead, there is no fear. There is want of nothing. There is no pain and no ego, no have-tos or shoulds. When I am dead, I have no worries about anything or anyone. There are no deadlines. It's total freedom and connectedness and bliss, but those words do not even compare to the feeling. It's something that cannot be described in words.

I now realize that there is nothing to fear. When I die again, I don't want any intervention. I just want to go. I am in no hurry to leave this life, but I'm not afraid to leave it, either. There may be more for me to do on this level, I guess, or I wouldn't keep coming back.

> *Chase's Unbeatable Advice:* Dying really isn't that bad. It's just the next phase of our consciousness. You just go to another place, a wonderful place, so don't fear it.

❋   BACK TO LIFE R$_x$ ❋

- Call your doctor as often as needed.
- Take your advocate, your iPod, a notebook, and a list of questions to your appointments.
- Get all the tests your doctor recommends, and ask for others you've read about.
- Schedule your appointments for the morning.
- Sign up for cardiac rehabilitation and go!

7

Step 5:
Make Love
to Your Partner Again

SEX IS ALL ABOUT FEELING GOOD. AS JAMIE AND I READIED FOR OUR first sexual experience after my surgery, however, I did not feel good about myself at all. I was embarrassed by how I looked, not only by my midline scar but also by my skinny body. I'd lost so much weight! I went from about 150 pounds to 130. I wasn't particularly sexy!

So many worries ran through my mind. *What if my heart rate goes up and I can't get it back down? What if I can't get an erection? What if I can't climax? What if I can't perform in a way that allows her to climax? What if she is not attracted to me anymore? What if I don't have the physical strength needed to perform?*

And there was the big one: *What if I die while we are having sex?*

I felt totally inadequate.

I was so afraid of failing that I talked about sex with my therapist before I talked about it with Jamie. My therapist advised me to practice alone first, so I could become confident about my ability to get and maintain an erection and to ejaculate—without killing myself off in the process.

What did I learn? Yes, my heart rate went up, as usual. Yes, I got sweaty. Yes, I felt anxious. Yes, I felt good on many levels. No, I didn't die.

It gave me the courage I needed to reclaim my sex life with my wife.

The Odds of Dying During Sex

In reality, making love to your partner probably will not trigger a heart attack. I know that now. To some extent, I knew it then, too. The odds of having a heart attack during sex—even if you've already suffered a heart attack—are only about twenty in one million.[1] Less than 1 percent of people who die from heart attacks do so during sex.[2] It makes a great scene in a movie, but it's just not all that common.

Indeed, you and I are much more likely to die in a car accident, from the collision, mind you.

It's one thing to know these statistics, though. It's another to truly believe them, and the only way to do that is to do what you most fear. You need to have sex.

And sex is important.

Sexual relations are good for you. Sex increases circulation and has been shown to improve cholesterol levels.[3] Sex reduces stress and improves sleep, both of which are extremely important for your heart. The hormone oxytocin released during lovemaking helps numb pain. A study of 914 men in South Wales, UK, determined that men who had sex most often (two or more times a week) were significantly less likely to die of heart disease than those who had sex less often (less than once a month).[4]

But You're Still Scared

So was I, and I'm a doctor who knows all the stats I just wrote by heart. No matter how strong you think you are, the diagnosis of heart disease takes your breath away, but it doesn't have to end your sex life.

If you decide to never be intimate again—because you are too scared—you'll become even more depressed about your heart disease. The loss of sexual intimacy will become one more loss that you must accept. You'll never be able to see yourself for what you really are—a sensual man or woman, one who deserves love, support, and adoration. We are sexual beings and sensual creatures. Loving and being loved define many of us. They are important.

There is no question that it takes time to garner the courage you need to make love to your partner again, but you really can do it. It will take time for you to become the person you once were in the bedroom, but you will become that person again. I'm living proof.

How do you know when you are ready? Sexual activity makes the heart work about as hard as it does while climbing two flights of stairs. If you can walk up that many stairs, you are probably strong and healthy enough to have sex.

Talk to your doctor, especially if you are worried. Your doctor can reduce your fears, which will go a long way to helping you enjoy the experience. Although it may be embarrassing to mention such problems to your

My husband was terrified of having sex. Whenever we talked about bringing sex back into our lives, he responded with the same question: "What if I die?" I was scared, too. It's not exactly romantic or exciting to be intimate with someone who has a huge midline scar on his chest. We both worried that, when the time came, sexual desire would evade us.

I knew our first sexual experience after the bypass was the most important. If it did not go well, each subsequent experience could become increasingly more difficult. So I took every precaution I could think of to ensure that we were both filled with sexual desire. I played soft music. I lit candles. Perhaps most important, I made sure to go slowly. We started with cuddling. I placed my head on his chest and listened to his heart. I told him, "Your heartbeat is so strong. I can hear it beating. It's so loud and so strong." Doing so helped us both relax. In fact, as soon as I made the comment, I saw Marc smile. Everything went smoothly after that, and it was a definite turning point in our relationship together and in Marc's continued recovery.

doctor, it's important to do so. Keep in mind that many heart disease patients experience sexual problems. You are not the only one. Chances are your doctor is not embarrassed by this topic at all.

Of course, this will only work if you have a warm, compassionate doctor with excellent bedside manner. If your physician is extremely competent but cold and standoffish, it's understandable that you might not feel comfortable asking questions about when, where, and how in the sexual department. You don't want the conversation to feel in any way, shape, or form like that initial birds-and-bees discussion you might have had many, many years ago with one of your parents!

If you determine that you just don't have the type of doctor who you can approach about such a touchy topic, then seek out the counsel of a therapist or other mental health professional. You might even consult a sex therapist. Make sure you find the warm, kind, compassionate person who allows you to feel comfortable talking about the topic.

Get Past the Fear

Making love to Jamie again was one of the most difficult issues I had to face after surgery. After surgery my sexual drive and appetite were nonexistent. I worried that I wouldn't be able to finish what I started. I worried that if I lost my erection, I would feel less than a man. I worried, "Will I be able to perform, and show Jamie that I love her?"

If this sounds all too familiar, then use the following advice to renew your sex life.

Explain how you feel. Your partner may be ready for sexual relations long before you are ready. Remind your partner that you are still attracted to him or her, but you just need more time to feel comfortable with sexual intercourse. Talk about when and under what circumstances you will be ready for intercourse. Plan the first time together, creating a specific scenario that you both find comfortable and appealing. Pick a day and a time to give it a try.

Change locations, if needed. This is important if you had a heart attack or angina pain while in your bedroom. You eventually can return to the bedroom for sex, but your first few encounters probably should be in another room until you get used to the experience and feel relaxed about it. You might even consider going to a hotel.

Masturbate. Masturbation will allow you to get used to the sensations of sex (the increased heart rate, for instance) without the extra anxiety of having to perform. Masturbation taught me that I was ready. It gave me the courage to talk with Jamie about planning the first time.

Set the scene. Make your environment as soothing and relaxing as possible. Light candles. Dim the lights. Play music. Think about it as that very first time you had intercourse with the person you loved so many years ago. Plan this second first time with the same detail and intensity.

Visualize the experience first. Lie down. Close your eyes. In your mind, see the entire sexual experience from beginning to end. Try to use all your senses. What do you see, hear, and feel? If you feel anxious as you think about this first encounter, focus on your breathing—taking five or so deep, full breaths—before returning to the visualization.

Hold a practice session. Once you've planned the first time, hold a dress rehearsal (or an undressing rehearsal, as the case may be). Put on the music. Get out the massage oil. Do everything leading up to the main event, and then stop. This will help build your confidence, ease your anxiety, and allow you to feel wanted and loved without forcing you to combat the fear of dropping dead at the same time.

Once you feel secure with the dress rehearsal, allow your partner to pleasure you (and vice versa) before moving on to the main event.

Shop for sexy lingerie (for female heart patients). Look for undergarments that artfully cover any part of your body that makes you feel self-conscious. For instance, a teddy that covers the chest might cover your scar and allow you to feel sexy.

Don't be afraid to try new things. If you are still very fatigued, your sexual desire just may not be what it once was. This is normal. Be patient and experiment with new ways to increase your desire. Perhaps you might ask your partner to wear lingerie (if you are a man). You might read or watch erotica together. Perhaps you can share sexual fantasies or even try a sex toy. Be open-minded and have fun!

And new positions. Certain positions—with you either on your back or on your side—will be easier for you during your recovery. For the time being, avoid being on top while supporting your body weight with your hands—the typical missionary position. This can increase blood pressure.

Do it in the morning. Morning sunlight helps fight depression, which will help you get in the mood. That light proves to you that you made it through yet another night. In the light of the day (a new day), you will feel fresh and more alive, and you'll have more courage and energy to push your limits.

Address emotional pain. Sadness, depression, and anxiety can all kill sexual desire. See Chapter 4 if depression is interfering with your sexual desire, especially if it persists beyond three months posttreatment.

Depression is very common with heart disease survivors. Don't allow it to go untreated. You may need talk therapy as well as prescription mood elevators.

Talk to your doctor about your medications. Some medicines used to treat heart disease can interfere with a man's ability to have an erection. Talk to your doctor about other alternatives or solutions. Again, you need a doctor you feel comfortable talking to about such issues.

If needed, talk to your doctor about Viagra and similar medicines. These medicines work by constricting the blood vessels, which slightly reduces the amount of blood flowing back to the heart. This should not be an issue if you've had surgery to fix your coronaries, though, so the medication should have little, if any, effect on your heart. It might provide a psychological benefit if your thoughts are preventing you from getting and maintaining an erection. Be sure to vet this through your cardiologist.

Talk to your gynecologist about contraception. If you are a young woman with heart disease, your doctor may advise you to stop taking oral contraceptives, as they can raise your risk of having a heart attack, especially if you smoke. You may want to investigate other forms of contraception, such as a diaphragm or condoms. If you are finished having children, consider asking your husband to undergo a vasectomy. Note: You could also investigate having your tubes tied, but I think the last thing you need after heart surgery is yet another surgery!

Similarly, you can talk to your gynecologist about any sexual issues you may be having.

Keep in mind that your first time may not go perfectly. You might not get all the way through the experience without stopping. You might become too scared, too tense, or too fatigued. You might not be able to maintain an erection. Any number of things might go wrong. It's very important to understand these issues as normal problems. Laugh about it. Move on. Try again. Sex is an important part of your being and an important part of your relationship with your partner. Keep trying. If needed, seek counseling from a sex therapist.

And here's something else you really need to know: It's okay if you cry. It really is. Jamie and I both cried after that first time. It was such a relief to know that this part of our lives was still intact.

❋ **BACK TO LIFE R$_x$** ❋

- Sex, as needed, when ready. Doctor's orders. It won't kill you. Trust me. I'm a doctor. I know.
- Think about it first.
- Then practice, alone.
- Then try it with your partner, in the morning, after setting the scene for romance.

---

* CHAPTER *

8

Step 6:
Embrace
Your Dinner Plate

IF YOU THINK THERE'S NO WAY YOU CAN PART WITH HIGH-FAT,
high-sugar, high-heart-attack-potential foods, all I can tell you is this: You
can. I know, because I did.

No one was more addicted to bad foods than I was. No one. My bad
eating habits started when I was a teenager, when I attended a prestigious
magnate school for boys in Philadelphia. This was the type of school that
only admitted near-genius kids, and it (and our parents) expected a lot
from us. There I was, at the same school as a young math whiz who was
so advanced that he was already teaching mathematics to college sopho-
mores at a nearby university. Another one of my classmates had already
written and published a book of poetry. It was the kind of place where one

could easily feel outclassed and outsmarted during homeroom. There was so much pressure to achieve.

To soothe my anxiety, I turned to food. I went to fast-food restaurants for burgers and fries, cheesesteak stands for the works, and ice cream parlors for sundaes. At diners I indulged in peach pie, lemon pie, and crumb cake. In college my bad eating habits continued. Every Friday night I celebrated the end of the week with chicken Parmesan that was drenched in cheese, followed by tiramisù. Then came medical school and more of the same. Each morning before class, I'd stop at a diner for orange juice (perhaps the only fruit serving I ever had), fried eggs, six pieces of bacon, fried potatoes, and toast slathered with butter. I'd go through jumbo-size chocolate bars by the dozen.

By the time I became a physician, I was an all-out stress eater, one who had no control whatsoever when sweets of any kind were around. I vividly remember my first job in St. Louis. Not only did I live on pizza, cakes, and ice cream, I had almost no self-control. On weekends I frequently took my children, Joshua and Jessica, to Winchell's doughnut shop. I asked them to pick out doughnuts for themselves for the next morning's breakfast. We always got two dozen.

But the doughnuts rarely if ever lasted through the night. Sometimes when my kids got up the following morning, they each got just one. Many other times they woke to discover that there were no doughnuts left. Their dad had eaten all of them. On these mornings my daughter would cry.

So, you see, I know just how attached you may be to certain foods. I've been there. I know all about that! Food serves as a powerful force in our lives. It fills us up. It gives us energy. It comforts us. It tastes good. Certain foods can even represent the gamut of emotions, from joy to sadness to guilt. They evoke memories of childhood and family.

I know about food temptation, but I also know this: These attachments can be broken. I'm living proof. Today I rarely, if ever, eat sweets. When I order dessert, I have just a taste, a thumbprint's worth. If the father who once ate his kids' doughnuts can find the willpower to consume only one bite of a dessert that no one else plans to eat, you can do it, too.

More important, it's probably not as difficult or onerous as you might suspect. Heart-healthy eating isn't the same thing as bland eating or joyless eating. You can eat for a healthy heart and still eat for flavor. You can enjoy every aspect of your eating experience without fearing that every molecule of the food you are eating will eventually clog your arteries.

You really can. I'm about to show you how.

Start by breaking your transition to heart-healthy eating into three phases or steps.

Phase I Eating

Phase 1 eating takes place during the initial weeks and months after your heart attack or surgery. During this time, you'll probably notice that your appetite just isn't what it used to be. You might not have an appetite at all. Much like a pregnant woman during her first trimester, you may even feel nauseous at the thought of eating or at the sight or smell of food. Your sense of taste may be diminished, too.

No one is really sure precisely why this happens. Some of the lack of appetite may stem from the anesthesia or from aftereffects of being hooked up to the heart-lung machine. If you are not yet moving your bowels regularly (which is a side effect of the surgery and of some types of pain medicines), you probably won't feel particularly hungry, either. Pain medicines, bed rest, and the fatigue induced from the surgery itself can also reduce your appetite and zest for eating.

All of those causes usually are temporary and lift within a few weeks. A longer-lasting cause of poor appetite, however, is depression. (Depression, by the way, can also cause you to gain an appetite. Everyone reacts to depression differently.)

When I got depressed after my surgery, I completely lost my appetite. I would look at the food—any food—and just could not muster up any enthusiasm for eating. Even Cheerios, once my favorite breakfast food, seemed gross to me. I just didn't want to eat. I tried to convince myself that I wasn't emaciated and that I did not look like Jamie's father. In reality, however, I was withering away. I could see my ribs. When I weighed in at 130, Jamie flipped out. As a comparison, I'm 150 now, and that's still pretty slim.

Every time I ate, I worried that the food I consumed would clog my arteries or cause a clot to form. I couldn't even eat chicken soup without worrying that some fat from the chicken might have made its way into the soup and would eventually kill me. For me eating seemed like a life-or-death proposition. If I wanted to live, I just wouldn't eat. If I wanted to die, I'd eat.

That thinking, of course, doesn't seem remotely rational to me now, but it did then. No wonder I had no appetite for so many weeks post-surgery!

I was also scared of gaining weight. The idea of eating made me nervous. As a health-conscious physician, I knew the research. I knew that every extra pound raised my risk for heart attack. The thing is, those were extra pounds above ideal body weight. I wasn't anywhere near ideal. At six feet tall and 130 pounds, I was underweight.

If any of this sounds remotely familiar to you, you need to understand that your mind is playing tricks on you. Your body knows that it needs food, but your mind is so sad about your condition that it just does not make it seem that any food (even your favorites) is worthwhile.

That's why Phase 1 is designed for one purpose and one purpose only: to get calories and nutrients into your body in the least upsetting way possible.

During Phase 1, eating is a relative term because much of what I suggest you consume will be liquid. You'll be doing more drinking and slurping than you'll be doing true eating.

Use these pointers:

- Stay away from gas-producing and acidic foods. The last thing you need when you have pain from your incision is a huge gas bubble or heartburn. If a food used to upset your stomach or produce heartburn before surgery, don't go near it during Phase 1. Common offenders include beans, onions, tomatoes and tomato sauce, orange juice, coffee, chocolate, and fatty foods (such as fried foods). Because most fruits and vegetables are hard to digest, you might also want to stay away from them for quite a while.

- Similarly, you want to stay away from spicy foods with a strong flavor. These are the foods that are most likely to make you feel nauseous. I loved spicy foods, but after surgery they were impossible to eat.

- Eat frequent, small meals. You may not be able to stomach the quantity of food you used to eat. Don't torture yourself. Have many small snacks instead of a few big meals. Not only will this reduce nausea, it's also good for your health. Research shows that frequent small meals help better stabilize blood sugar levels, improve energy, and reduce cholesterol levels. You'll feel better and become healthier at the same time.

- Relax before meals. I learned the importance of this practice quite by accident. I'd been having trouble walking outdoors without feeling anxious, so my psychologist suggested I take a small amount of Valium (a tranquilizer) before going for a walk. One day I did. Jamie and I walked down to a Chinese restaurant. Suddenly, for the first time in four weeks, I had an appetite! I ordered wonton soup and chicken and vegetables. Food tasted good again, and I realized that anxiety over the idea of eating was killing my appetite.

- Use Ensure between meals or as a meal, since it tastes good and is easily digested.

    You don't necessarily have to take a Valium in order to develop an appetite, though. Just do some deep breathing, the same type of breathing I suggested in Chapter 4 to help relax. Slowly bring the air deep into your lungs, filling your abdomen and rib cage. Then slowly exhale. Do this a few times, until you feel relaxed.

- Phase 3 will help you evolve into a heart-healthy eater. Don't worry about eating heart-healthy right now. Just eat. Eat any food that turns you on to eating. You need to get your strength back. If you want a steak, have it. If you want ice cream, have it. Your goal is to eat anything that you find palatable. Your mind might fight you, but it is important to eat whatever you can get down.

- Eat at the table and not lying in bed or on the couch. Eating while seated will help prevent heartburn. And you will be more likely to linger and eat more if you are in the dining room, and particularly if you are eating with the rest of your family. Make eating as pleasant and enjoyable as possible. Light candles. Set the table. Listen to soft music. Enjoy every part of the experience. I found that whenever I lit candles and played classical music during a meal, eating felt like a mellow, worthwhile experience.

- Go liquid. Soups, smoothies, and soft foods (applesauce, Jell-O, pudding, and yogurt) are ideal during this phase. Check out the Phase 1 recipes (pages 249–254) for inspiration. Also, keep supplemental drinks, such as Ensure, on hand at all times. Ensure provides calories and taste at a minimum cost. Use it to make a smoothie with nonfat ice cream or frozen fruit.

- Choose foods that bring you comfort. Have the soup that your mom used to make when you were home sick as a child, for instance. Choose foods that evoke calming, happy memories.

- Invest in a blender so you and your caregiver can puree soups and smoothies to your liking.

Phase 2 Eating

Advance to Phase 2 whenever you feel ready. The time for Phase 2 will vary from person to person. You might be ready within just a few days of surgery, or it might take many weeks. You'll know you are ready when you no longer fear food and when you feel a hankering for more-substantive meals.

Phase 2 is an intermediate phase, designed to get you used to eating semisolids and solids. I am a big proponent of comfort foods during Phase 2. That's right, we're talking macaroni and cheese, meat loaf, and mashed potatoes. Although such foods may not qualify as the healthiest foods on the planet, you are still getting your strength back and still getting used to eating. Comfort foods will allow you to do just that. Check our Phase 2 recipes (pages 254–267) for ideas on how to make over traditional comfort food classics such as macaroni and cheese into meals that are comforting, delicious, and heart-healthy.

As with Phase 1, you probably still want to stay away from very spicy and flavorful foods during this phase, especially if you are still experiencing any nausea or chest discomfort. While in Phase 2, consume anything from Phase 1, plus the following foods:

Oatmeal: Buy lots of different types of flavored oatmeal, experimenting until you find a flavor that makes you want to eat. You can even add cinnamon (which has been shown to help control blood glucose) and raisins (also good for you). When I added cinnamon and raisins to oatmeal, it reminded me of eating a favorite cake or cookie.

Potatoes and other root vegetables: Baked potatoes, sweet potatoes, winter squash (see recipes, pages 257, 265–267), and mashed potatoes are all great options.

Heartier soups and stews: Try chili, stew, and other chunkier, meatier soups than you did in Phase 1. Check out Jamie's Vegetarian Chili (page 259).

Comfort foods: Go for macaroni and cheese (see recipe, page 260), grilled cheese (tip: use low-fat cheese, whole-grain bread, and Benecol instead of butter), scrambled eggs or egg whites, turkey meat loaf (see recipe, page 263), and other hearty comfort foods.

Desserts: You're still getting your strength back, so eat what you love. Many desserts can be just as delicious as they are good for you, too. See the desserts section on pages 274–277—we've included many delicious favorites with a heart-healthy twist.

Continually add more and more foods as you get back your strength.

Try to make your plate as colorful as possible and use as many different textures as possible. For instance, once you feel ready, try our Quick and Easy Fajitas (page 261). They contain mushrooms and peppers, which are great vegetables for your heart and are the perfect size for a small appetite. The more varied your plate, the more appetite you'll have to eat what's on your plate. So mix crunchy foods with smooth foods, red foods with yellow foods and green foods, and heavy foods with light foods.

Phase 3 Eating

By Phase 3, you will be feeling stronger. Your appetite should be back, and you may mistakenly get cocky, thinking that your heart surgery gave you a free "get out of food-jail card." Instead of eating a heart-healthy diet, you pile on the fries, doughnuts, and burgers, assuming your bypassed arteries just bought you twenty more years no matter how poorly you eat.

For example, about six months after my surgery, I was at an Italian restaurant with two other doctors. Two of us had had open-heart surgery. One talked about how it had added another ten years to his life. He ordered steak and pasta, and he spread butter on his bread.

I don't know what he was thinking. He was a doctor! He should have known better!

This type of unhealthy eating is just a form of denial, and denial is a form of repressed fear. A bad diet will undermine any drug or surgical procedure.

It's very important to follow a heart-healthy diet. The foods you eat can either contribute to heart disease (not to mention cancer, diabetes, and other health problems) by clogging your arteries, raising your blood pressure, and increasing the inflammation that triggers harmful blood clots.

Or they can contribute to long-lasting great health by feeding your arteries the nutrients they need to heal, reducing your cholesterol, lowering your blood pressure, and giving you the energy you need to practice other heart-healthy habits such as exercise.

Heart-healthy eating does not have to be synonymous with boredom, though. Plenty of delicious, flavorful foods are also incredibly good for your heart and blood vessels. Also, many foods that have gotten a bad reputation—such as olives, avocados, and even chocolate—are actually good for you. Others can easily be made heart-healthy with just a few simple tweaks. I'll show you how.

Eat These Foods, Live Longer

Most heart-healthy foods are Mother Nature's best inventions. They grow on trees or bushes or in the ground. They are not man-made.

Water. Have at least eight glasses a day. Carry water with you at all times, as I still do. Sip from it often. The water you drink helps add fluid to your blood. When your blood is more watery and less viscous, it's easier for your heart to pump blood throughout your body.

Fish. I eat fish two or three times a week and recommend that you do the same. Fatty cold-water fish such as salmon contains high amounts of a type of heart-healthy fat called omega-3 fatty acids. Research shows that eating fish regularly (and taking fish-oil capsules) can reduce your risk of developing or worsening heart disease by reducing levels of triglycerides (harmful fats in the bloodstream), lowering blood pressure, reducing the formation of blood clots, and stabilizing your heart rhythm.[1] Try to eat fish at least twice a week, but choose low-mercury-containing varieties whenever possible. Mercury, PCBs, and other industrial contaminants have infiltrated our oceans and waterways. These contaminants raise your risk for heart disease and other health problems. The fish with the highest levels of these contaminants tend to be larger and live a long time. They include shark, swordfish, king mackerel, and tilefish. To optimize omega-3 fatty acids and minimize mercury ingestion, focus on canned light tuna, wild salmon, and sardines.

Avocados. Yes, they are high in calories. Yes, they are high in fat. Yes, they taste phenomenal when made into guacamole. And yes, they are good for your heart! Rich in fiber and heart-healthy monounsaturated fat, avocados may actually help lower cholesterol. In one Mexican study, people who ate an avocado every day for a week saw a 17 percent drop in cholesterol levels, with LDLs (the bad type) plummeting and HDLs (the good type) climbing. Avocados are also rich in a substance called beta-sitosterol, which also has been shown to reduce cholesterol levels.

Olive oil and olives. Olives are rich in heart-healthy monounsaturated fat and in the antioxidant vitamin E, which is important in preventing cholesterol from oxidizing. They also contain heart-healthy plant chemicals called polyphenols and flavonoids, which reduce inflammation. Use olives as a flavorful topping on fish and chicken. They also make a great, satisfying snack. Or add them to salads for a little extra zing. Jamie keeps olive oil in a spritz bottle and uses it to dress salads and add flavor to other dishes.

Nuts. Like avocados and olives, nuts are also high in fat—but, again, it's the good kind. Most of the fat in nuts is either monounsaturated or polyunsaturated, and many studies have linked an increased consumption of nuts with a decreased incidence of heart disease. In the Iowa Women's Health Study of thousands of women, for instance, women who ate nuts more than four times a week were 40 percent less likely to die of heart disease than women who ate nuts less often. In a separate study done at Harvard, men who

> ### ▣ YOU CAN'T BEAT THIS ADVICE! ▣
>
> Mash up avocado and use it as a spread in place of butter or mayonnaise.

ate nuts two or more times a week also reduced their risk of sudden cardiac death. In addition to healthful fat, nuts are a rich source of fiber, heart-healthy plant chemicals, and antioxidants such as vitamin E and selenium. Eat up to 1.5 ounces a day, which amounts to roughly ⅓ cup almonds or walnuts. You could also try a nut-and-dried-fruit mixture. Dried fruits taste incredible, and are good for you, too.

Fruits and vegetables. Fruits and vegetables are probably the best foods for your overall health. They are loaded with health-promoting plant chemicals such as flavonoids, lycopene, lutein, and various carotenoids. These plant chemicals work as antioxidants to scavenge harmful free radicals before they can damage your blood vessels. A Serbian study that tracked the health outcomes of 290 cardiac patients and about 200 healthy people determined that people with heart disease tended to consume fewer vegetables. People who ate vegetables just once a week were three times more likely to develop heart disease compared to people who ate them at least once a day and were four times as likely to get heart disease compared to people who ate several servings a day.[2]

The minerals in fruits and vegetables—especially potassium—may help reduce blood pressure. And because vegetables are rich in fiber and water and low in calories, they fill you up on fewer calories, helping you maintain a healthy weight. Most experts recommend that you consume at least five daily servings of fruits and vegetables, with some going as high as eight to ten.

When choosing fruits and vegetables:

- Aim for a variety. The more types you eat, the greater the variety of antioxidants you consume. Antioxidants seem to have different functions in the body, with some working to reduce heart disease and others helping save your eyesight, fight cancer, and perform other miraculous tasks. Some increase the effectiveness of others, too, so a variety is key.
- Consume brightly colored varieties. Antioxidants are often found in the pigments that give fruits and vegetables their bright colors. Bright yellow, red, purple, and dark green fruits and vegetables are much healthier for you than paler types. For instance, dark leafy greens contain more antioxidants than paler iceberg lettuce.
- Choose lower-sugar fruits. Northern fruits (berries, melons, apples, pears, and peaches) contain less sugar than tropical fruits (pineapple, bananas, and mangoes) and tend to produce a more even rise in blood sugar. If you have diabetes or prediabetes, stick with nontropical varieties.
- Eat the whole fruit. It's better to eat an orange—which has fiber—than to drink commercially prepared orange juice, which has very little fiber and more added sugar. In general, the less processed any food is, the better it is for you. If you love orange juice, it's worth buying oranges and squeezing them yourself.

Whole grains. Just like fruits and vegetables, many grains contain heart-healthy plant chemicals. In fact, a Wake Forest University study of more than 149,000 men and women determined that people who consumed more whole grains (2½ servings a day) reduced their risk of heart disease by 21 percent compared to people who had just .2 servings a day.[3] A diet rich in whole grains has been shown to help steady blood sugar, improve the health of your blood vessels, and reduce cholesterol.

But it's really important to eat the *whole* grain. Most flour-based foods are made from just one small part of a grain. Rice, wheat, and other grains contain three parts.

1. **The bran.** This outermost covering of the grain contains fiber and protein, certain vitamins and minerals, and healing plant chemicals. Fiber might help reduce cholesterol by forming a gel-like mass in your intestine and slowing the absorption of sugar and fat into your bloodstream. Oat bran in particular has been shown to lower cholesterol, which is why whole slow-cooking oats should be a big part of your recovery plan.
2. **The germ.** This is the food source for the seed inside the grain. It contains heart-healthy plant chemicals, antioxidants, vitamin E, and B vitamins.
3. **The endosperm.** This is all that's left after a grain is refined. It has little to no fiber, antioxidants, minerals, and plant chemicals. It's basically vitamin-vacant starch.

It's important to consume grains that are as minimally processed as possible. For instance, you'll find some instant varieties of brown rice and oatmeal. These foods cook faster, in part because the grain has been mashed and processed into smaller bits. Yet the larger and more intact the grain, the longer it takes for the intestine to break it down. Instant oatmeal, for instance, is still "whole." It contains all parts of the grain, but it has been pulverized. This essentially predigests the food for you. Because there is more surface area for enzymes in your intestine to work on, they break down these pulverized grains faster, allowing glucose to enter your bloodstream at a quicker rate.

In earlier phases, I suggested that you consume flavored oatmeal. That was largely because I just wanted you to eat, and these types of oatmeal are more palatable for most people. Now that you are in Phase 3, it's important to try to transition into eating less-processed whole grains. Opt for slow-cooking steel-cut oats, brown rice, and other grains over their instant counterparts.

Chocolate. See? Healthy eating really isn't that bad, now, is it? Chocolate is indeed a heart-healthy food. The cocoa in chocolate may reduce blood pressure by helping the body better process nitric oxide. Cocoa is also rich in flavonoids, a heart-healthy plant chemical that prevents harmful blood clots and keeps fat in the bloodstream from clogging your arteries.

It's important to choose dark chocolate with a high cocoa content. This type of chocolate is not only rich in those heart-protective flavonoids, it also has more fiber and less sugar than other types of chocolate. If you have diabetes, you probably can eat small amounts of this type of chocolate and not see your blood sugar skyrocket. Look for bars that are 75 percent cocoa or higher, and indulge in just two squares or fewer at a time.

Wine. Alcohol—whether from wine, beer, or spirits—seems to prevent fat from getting stuck on the lining of your arteries. Wine and dark beer also contain protective plant compounds that act as antioxidants to protect the lining of your arteries from damage.

Keep in mind that medicines you may be taking may intensify the effects of alcohol. I learned this the hard way when I was on a business trip. I had two drinks during dinner. Later that night, I got back to my hotel and felt like my room was spinning! I was sweaty, disoriented, and very scared. Now I hold myself to just one drink, and I sip it very slowly. I recommend you do the same. Consume alcohol with meals (not on an empty stomach) and keep it to one daily serving: 12 ounces of beer, 4 ounces of wine, or a 1.5-ounce shot.

Margarine made from plant sterols. Sterols are fats from plants that prevent the body from absorbing cholesterol from the food you eat. They also inhibit your liver from making cholesterol. They are naturally found in many plant foods such as avocados, nuts, and soybeans, but you'd have to eat sixteen avocados a day for three weeks to consume enough of these substances to affect your cholesterol levels. That's where sterol-fortified products come in. These substances have now been added to many processed foods, including margarine. One brand, Benecol, has been extensively studied and shown to reduce cholesterol, enough to drop heart disease risk by 25 percent when used as a substitute for regular margarine or butter.[4] I use it in place of butter on whole-grain toast each morning. It's a delicious butter substitute that has helped me maintain a low cholesterol reading.

What Not to Eat

Reduce your consumption of these foods and substances:

Refined starches. For many years we were told that carbs were good, that they were the main fuel source of the body. This is still true, but not

To make sure you are really getting a whole-grain product, look on the list of ingredients and use the following to decide whether or not the ingredients are whole or refined.

Whole-Grain Ingredients

- Whole-wheat flour
- Buckwheat
- Bulgur
- Millet
- Wild rice
- Brown rice
- Oats
- Wheat berries

Not Necessarily Whole-Grain Ingredients

- Wheat flour
- Semolina
- Durum wheat

Refined-Grain Ingredients

- Enriched flour
- Degerminated cornmeal

To make choices easier for consumers, the Whole Grains Council allows companies to place a stamp on their products. If you see a 100% stamp on a product, it means that all the grains used to make the product are whole grains.

all carbs are good for you. Your body converts carbohydrates into blood glucose, and your cells use glucose to create energy. If you ingest more carbohydrate—either from starchy foods such as potatoes or from sugar-sweetened foods such as candy—than your cells need at any given time, the excess is converted into glycogen and stored in your liver and muscle cells. Your liver and muscle cells, however, can only store so much glycogen, so if you eat too much carbohydrate at once, at least some of it gets converted into triglycerides (a type of fat), which can raise your risk of heart disease in two ways:

1. Triglycerides float around in the bloodstream and can directly contribute to the clogging of your arteries.
2. Triglycerides eventually are stored inside your fat cells. Weight gain raises your risk of heart disease.

You raise the risk of your body converting the carbohydrate you eat into fat when you consume refined carbs that digest rapidly. The faster your body breaks down these foods, the faster glucose enters your bloodstream. You can slow the absorption of carbohydrates into your bloodstream by consuming whole-grain carbs that contain decent amounts of fiber.

Sugar. It's bad for your heart for the same reason refined starch is bad for your heart. Cut back on sugar by:

- Eliminating or diluting soft drinks and fruit juices with seltzer.
- Eating sweets after a meal, when you have more control, and never on an empty stomach. Rather than eating a full dessert portion, use the three-bite rule, and savor every bite. You'll notice that the third bite does not taste as good as the first.

- Eating the same sweet treat every day. You'll grow accustomed to the taste, so you'll have an easier time sticking with and feeling satisfied with a smaller portion.
- Eating tempting foods only when you are away from home. You'll eat less ice cream, for instance, if you have to drive or walk to get it, rather than just go to your freezer.
- Hiding tempting foods. Studies show that people automatically eat less of certain foods if they can't see them or if it takes a lot of work to break into them. Clip sweet treats closed and wrap them in foil. Put the foil in a zip-top bag and the bag in a box that you tape closed.
- Finding low-fat packaged foods that do not substitute sugar for fat. Pretzels are a good low-fat substitute for potato chips, but low-fat cookies are not a good substitute for high-fat cookies, due to the addition of sugar. The same is true for low-fat peanut butter.
- Opting for the real thing over fake sugar. A little real sugar in moderation is okay. Sugar substitutes contain all sorts of chemicals that may not be good for you.

Saturated fat. Found in fatty animal products, this type of fat raises cholesterol levels. The National Heart, Lung, that and Blood Institute recommends that you consume fewer than 7 percent of your calories from saturated fat. You can cut back on saturated fat by switching to nonfat dairy products and sticking to lean cuts of meat. Eat red meat (which tends to be fatty) rarely, and when you do, stick to the leaner cuts, such as sirloin and top loin. Most of the fat in poultry is in the skin and just underneath it, so stick with skinless chicken and turkey. I never eat chicken or turkey skin these days, and I keep all meat portions to the size of my palm. One exception to this rule is eggs. Although all the fat and cholesterol is housed in the yolk, the yolk also houses most of the nutrition. For example, egg yolks are a rich source of vitamin A and heart-healthy carotenoids.

Trans fats. These man-made fats were invented to increase the shelf life of processed foods. Trans fats are made by hydrogenating liquid oils. They raise levels of the bad LDL cholesterol and lower levels of the good HDL cholesterol. Try to eliminate them from your diet. You'll find trans fats in any processed food that lists the words "hydrogenated" or "partially hydrogenated" on the label. Food manufacturers are required by law to list the grams of trans fats on their labels. Only buy foods that list them as zero.

Sodium. Sodium causes the body to retain water, which makes your heart work harder to pump blood. If you are on diuretics, any sodium you eat will counter these medications. Consume no more than 2400 milligrams of sodium (roughly 1 teaspoon of salt) a day. Cut back on sodium by:

- Substituting Mrs. Dash or another spice for the saltshaker. Many spices and herbs not only lend a wonderful flavor to your food, they also help improve your health. Most spices contain powerful health-promoting antioxidants. Cinnamon, for instance, has been shown to help control blood sugar and reduce dangerous blood clots. Ginger may help relax blood vessels and stimulate blood flow. Turmeric, chiles, and sage all reduce heart-disease-causing inflammation. Chiles may also help reduce blood cholesterol and triglyceride levels.
- Cutting back on processed foods. Nearly 77 percent of the sodium in a typical person's diet comes from prepared and processed foods. When you do purchase these foods, look for the words "sodium free," "very low sodium," "reduced sodium," "light in sodium," or "unsalted" on the label.

Not all fat is bad for you. In fact, some types of fat are quite good for your health. Use this cheat sheet to know your fats.

Monounsaturated fats

Effects: Increase HDL (the good cholesterol), lower LDL (the bad cholesterol).

Types of foods: Olive oil, canola oil, peanut oil, avocados, nuts.

Polyunsaturated fats

Effects: Lower LDL (the bad cholesterol).

Types of foods: Sunflower seeds, walnuts, and most vegetable oils.

Omega-3 fatty acids

Effects: Improve health by stabilizing heart rhythm, boosting mood, preventing blood clots, and reducing cholesterol.

Types of foods: Fatty fish such as salmon, flaxseed, and walnuts.

Saturated fats

Effects: Raise LDL (the bad cholesterol) and total cholesterol, raising the risk for heart disease.

Types of foods: Fatty cuts of pork, beef, and lamb, poultry with skin, and fatty dairy products, including butter. If you occasionally indulge in fatty meats, keep your portion to the size of your palm.

Trans fats

Effects: Lower HDLs (the good cholesterol), and increase LDLs (the bad cholesterol).

> **Types of foods:** Margarine, vegetable shortening, fried foods, pro-
> cessed baked goods, partially hydrogenated oils, or hydrogenated
> vegetable oil. Only purchase packaged foods that list a zero next
> to the words "trans fat" on the Nutrition Facts label.

- Avoiding foods that list baking soda (sodium bicarbonate), baking powder (unless it's a sodium-free variety), soy sauce, nitrate, disodium phosphate, monosodium glutamate, and sodium within the first three ingredients. Canned foods, frozen dinners, commercially prepared soups, and condiments generally contain high amounts of sodium. Look for better, fresher choices.

Do you have to eliminate these foods from your diet? No! Just follow Marc's number one heart-healthy rule:

Eat to Live 98 percent of the time. When you Eat to Live, you fuel your body with fruits, vegetables, whole grains, beans, and lean protein your heart and body need for optimal health. These foods help you live longer.

Live to Eat the other 2 percent of the time. When you Live to Eat, you consume those tasty foods we all love that are not necessarily great for your heart. When you indulge, use this advice.

- Eat unhealthy foods after you've eaten healthy foods. Certain components of healthy foods—such as fiber—can reduce the disease-promoting wallop of not-so-healthy foods by slowing the absorption of glucose into your bloodstream and possibly even trapping some of the fat from food, preventing it from being absorbed at all. So if you want indulge in a dessert, do so, but have a salad and/or lean protein first.

- Share indulgence foods. Split that steak or dessert with your spouse. Jamie and I do this all the time, so we can each have a small taste of a treasured food. It helps us both enjoy the flavor of certain fatty foods while sticking to a reasonable portion.
- Go for a walk afterward. Moderate exercise helps the body more easily process the fat from the food you eat, so less of it is as likely to end up stuck to the sides of your arteries. It really works.

The Back-to-Life Diet

Rather than three big meals, try to eat five smaller meals. This helps with appetite in the beginning, but it also might help reduce blood cholesterol and blood sugar levels long term. When creating meals, always try to balance them with some protein (chicken, fish, eggs), a fruit or vegetable, and a healthy grain or starch (beans, brown rice, sweet potato, whole-grain bread).

Each day choose foods from the following food groups:[5]

5 to 10 colorful fruits and vegetables

1 fruit serving = 1 medium whole fruit (size of a tennis ball) or ½ cup cut fruit

1 vegetable serving = 1 cup leafy greens or ½ cup chopped cooked vegetables

4 to 8 ounces lean organic protein foods

4 ounces = palm-of-your-hand-size serving of game meat, chicken, fish, extra-lean beef, or shellfish

Two weekly servings should be fish.

1 to 3 servings high-fiber whole grains and legumes

1 serving = 1 slice bread, ½ cup cereal, pasta, beans, lentils, quinoa

1 to 3 servings healthful fat

1 serving = 1 tablespoon oil, one-eighth of an avocado, 8 large olives, 1.5 ounces nuts

1 to 2 servings high-calcium foods

1 serving = 1 cup nonfat or low-fat milk, 1.5 ounces low-fat or part-skim cheese, 6 ounces low-fat or nonfat yogurt

1 alcoholic drink 2 to 3 times a week (optional)

The Eat-to-Live Grocery List

Keep your pantry and kitchen stocked with the following staples.

Phase I

Ensure or a similar liquid meal-replacement product

Low-sodium chicken stock

Chicken breasts

Extra-lean ground beef or ground turkey breast

Fresh herbs, spices, and flavorings for soups: ginger, garlic, scallions

Mrs. Dash and other salt-free seasoning mixes

White vinegar

Vegetables for soups: carrots, onions, celery

Eggs, preferably omega-3 enriched

Progresso bean soup, low-sodium variety

Low-sodium chicken soup

Fat-free yogurt

Skim milk

Nonfat ice cream

Nonfat cream cheese

Nonfat cottage cheese

Fat-free Jell-O pudding

Cool Whip (nonfat)

Ice pops

Frozen fruit (strawberries, peaches, mangos) for smoothies

Fudge bars (100 calories or fewer per bar)

Spray oil such as Pam

Olive oil

Benecol

Whey protein powder for smoothies

Phase 2

Everything from Phase 1, plus:

Flavored instant oatmeal

Corn tortillas

Sweet potatoes and/or winter squash

Baking potatoes

Whole-grain pasta

Brown rice

Wild rice

Barley

Quinoa

Whole-grain bread

Dark chocolate

All-purpose flour

Whole-wheat flour

Cornmeal

Olive oil

Lean meat

Fish

Canned light tuna

Reduced-fat cheese slices

Phase 3

Everything from Phases 1 and 2, plus:

Steel-cut oats

High-fiber breakfast cereal

Tomato sauce

Tomato paste

Diced tomatoes

Canned beans

Tree nuts (almonds, walnuts, pistachios)

Wide assortment of fresh and frozen vegetables

Salad greens and other vegetables

Fresh fruit

Hummus

Dark chocolate

How to Read a Label

I didn't pay much attention to food labels before my bypass. Now I read every single one of them because I know that I am what I eat. I also know that advertisers do a very good job of making many not-so-healthy foods seem healthy. Why do you think certain sugar-coated breakfast cereals contain the word "fruit" in their name, even though there isn't a single molecule of fruit in the cereal? Because it makes the cereal sound healthy.

How can you avoid being duped? Before you buy any new packaged food, check out the Nutrition Facts label. Look for:

- The serving size and the servings per container. If you eat more than the listed serving size, you are eating more calories, fat, sugar, and everything else that the package lists.
- The grams of total fat, saturated fat, and trans fat. Ideally, you want the number next to "trans fat" to be a zero. You want the amount of saturated fat to be as low as possible, too, preferably under 2 grams per serving.
- The milligrams of sodium. You want to consume no more than 2,400 milligrams a day.
- The amounts of fiber, vitamins, and minerals. If these are all zeros, you are looking at a box of junk food. Skip it!

Also, know that the certain phrases on food packaging are designed to make you think the food is healthy, but really mean nothing. Take the phrase "made from whole grains." This just means that the product started out with whole grains, but little to none may actually have made their way into the product after processing. Food manufacturers can use this claim, but they are not required to state precisely how much (or how little) whole grains are actually in the product. The same is true for "made with real fruit" and "made with vegetables." Same with "natural" and "all natural." When you see claims like this, trust your gut. If you are looking at a piece of candy and the label says "made with real fruit," trust that little voice that mutters, "This is too good to be true." Second, look at the list of ingredients. The ingredients that appear first are present in a food in greater amounts than ingredients that appear last. If fruit is listed first? Great! The food might actually be good for you. If it's listed last? Not so much.

How to Eat Out

We live in New York City, which means one thing: We eat out a lot. You can still Eat to Live at restaurants. Use these tips and the corresponding ordering guide. Many of these eating lessons I learned from going to the Canyon Ranch spa, which I truly believe helped delay the event approximately ten to twelve years.

- Feel empowered to get what you want. Ask many questions and make special requests. Tell the waitstaff that you are "on a special diet" and can only eat low-fat foods that are baked or boiled without extra fat or oil. If the waitstaff won't help you, ask to speak to a manager or the chef. This is life or death. If they don't honor your requests, don't go back.
- Eat at the same restaurants a lot. The waitstaff will get to know you. Eventually you will not have to ask for the sauce on the side and no butter. They will remember you and do it automatically.
- Do not dine with people who try to get you to go off your special diet. It's just not worth the angst. If you are out with a large group of people and feel embarrassed to make special requests in front of others, pull the waiter over somewhere else in the restaurant so you can have your requests met.
- Look for appetizers like hummus, olives, salads, and warm, broth-based soups so you can fill up and are less likely to get a wandering eye for fatty menu options. It will also help you automatically eat less.
- Beware of soups. Ask a lot of questions before ordering to find out what's in the soup. Thick soups generally contain butter and cream, and broth-based soups are notoriously rich in salt. Other high-salt

foods are pickles (and anything that comes pickled), cocktail sauce, smoked foods, teriyaki sauce, soy sauce, and anything served au jus.

- Always get sauce on the side. Most restaurant sauces are loaded with fat, sugar, and salt. If you ask for sauce on the side and the food comes with sauce on it, send it back to the kitchen.
- Ask for your food to be prepared with olive oil instead of butter.
- Ask for olive oil at the table instead of butter.
- Get salad dressing on the side. Dip your fork in the dressing before piercing the salad rather than spooning or pouring the dressing directly on top. You'll use much less dressing this way.
- Use a napkin to blot pizza and other foods that look like they have a lot of grease.
- Ask for skim or low-fat milk and other dairy products to be substituted for any dairy that might come with the meal.
- Know that foods prepared the following ways tend to be lower in fat: baked, broiled, grilled, poached, roasted, and steamed. Foods prepared the following ways tend to be higher in fat: fried, sautéed, au

When we order pizza, we ask the kitchen to go light on the dough. In other words, we ask for a wafer-thin crust. Then we load it up with grilled chicken and veggies, and we stay clear of fried and greasy toppings like eggplant and extra cheese.

gratin, basted, braised, buttered, creamed, escalloped, pan-roasted, and stewed.

- Share your order, especially huge meals like steaks. When we don't share a meal (because we could not agree and finally decided to order two different entrées), we ask the kitchen to wrap half of each entrée right away—before it ever makes its way to the table—and we have it for lunch the next day. This is a great way to consume smaller portions.

Use these ordering suggestions when dining at the following types of restaurants.

Breakfast Diners

- Whole-grain or high-fiber breakfast cereal with skim milk. My favorites are Cheerios and Shredded Wheat.
- Fat-free or low-fat yogurt with fruit
- Oatmeal
- Veggie omelet
- Whole-grain pancakes
- English muffin and egg sandwich—substitute a tomato for the cheese and hold the butter.

Cajun

- Boiled crawfish, shrimp, or seafood
- Turkey or roast beef po'boy sandwich (on whole-grain bread if you can get it, or lose the bread)
- Red beans and rice (brown rice if you can get it). Note: Beware of most other Cajun side dishes. Most are high in sodium and fat.
- Jambalaya

Chinese

- Chicken or shrimp with steamed vegetables (sauce on the side)
- Hot and sour soup
- Wonton soup
- Steamed vegetable dumplings
- Steamed brown rice with tofu, sauce on the side

French

- Steamed mussels
- Crudités (raw cut vegetables)
- Pureed clear vegetable soup, such as pureed carrot or squash soup. Make sure it's prepared without cream or butter. Don't be afraid to ask.
- Boiled fish—squeeze fresh lemon or lime for added flavor.
- Small, 6-ounce steak served au poivre, split with your dining companion
- Fruit for dessert

Greek

- Dolmas (rice wrapped with grape leaves)
- Tzatziki, hummus, or baba ghanoush
- Shish kebab
- Grilled octopus or squid
- Whole fish
- Plaki

Indian

- Papadam
- Chicken or beef tikka
- Chicken, fish, or beef tandoori
- Vegetable or dal curry
- Shish kebab

Italian

- Minestrone soup
- Pasta fagioli soup
- Roasted peppers
- Grilled vegetables
- Broiled fish, with a side of tomato sauce for flavor (use only 2 to 3 tablespoons of the sauce).
- Chicken or fish marsala (with mushrooms and olive oil, and no butter)
- Veal or chicken paillard, grilled

Japanese

- Edamame (ask them not to add the usual salt).
- Miso soup
- Sushi (made with brown rice if possible)
- Chicken yakitori
- Half order of beef negimaki

Mexican

- Grilled shrimp
- Grilled fish
- Grilled chicken breast
- Beans with rice (brown if available)
- Chicken fajitas (ask that they be prepared with minimal oil, and skip the cheese and sour cream).
- Taco salad (do not eat the shell).
- Salsa
- Chicken or beef enchiladas, minus the cheese and sauce

Steakhouse

- Mixed green salad
- Grilled asparagus, broccoli, or squash
- Flank steak or petite filet mignon, smallest serving possible—add garlic and freshly ground pepper for flavor (a serving the size of your fist)

Heart-Healthy Supplements

I recommend you take the following supplements. Talk about each of them with your doctor first, to make sure they do not counter or overly accentuate the effects of prescription medications you might be taking. Please remember, these supplements are just that, and are to be treated as companions to prescription drugs. To me, taking them as supplements makes sense for your heart health. Daily aspirin, however, is mandatory.

Aspirin. As it turns out, aspirin does much more than numb pain. It blocks an enzyme called cyclooxygenase, which is needed for the body to produce the prostaglandins that cause inflammation. This helps thin your blood and reduce the formation of harmful blood clots. Results of the Women's Heart Study determined that taking 100 milligrams of aspirin daily can drop your risk of stroke by 17 percent. Research shows that a daily aspirin also prevents the recurrence of heart attack, angina, and stroke. Note: Don't drink alcohol if you are taking aspirin.

Coenzyme Q10 (CoQ10). This substance is naturally found in a part of human cells called the mitochondria. This energy compartment of the cell is where most of the harmful cell reactions take place. It's like a big furnace that generates a lot of heat and has lots of sparks (called free radicals) flying every which way. CoQ10 both helps create cell energy and extinguish those free radical sparks before they can land on something important, such as a cell membrane or piece of DNA, and damage it. As a result, CoQ10 helps keep cells throughout your body healthy.

CoQ10 might prevent heart disease by improving energy production in cells, inhibiting blood clots, and acting as an antioxidant that protects both the heart muscle and the lining of arteries. It may also help reduce blood pressure and improve blood-sugar control. Certain drugs used to treat heart disease may lower levels of this important enzyme, making supplementation a must. Talk to your doctor to determine whether this supplement is right for you.

B complex. The B vitamins folic acid, B_6, and B_{12} help keep homocysteine, an amino acid, from damaging the lining of your blood vessels. They break down this harmful metabolic by-product into a harmless substance that the body can excrete. A study done at the University of Wisconsin determined that high homocysteine levels were associated with heart disease, and that optimal levels of B vitamins helped lower homocysteine.[6] Harvard's School of Public Health research shows that B vitamins may halve heart disease risk in women.

You can consume B vitamins from your food, but you probably are not getting enough. As you age, you lose your ability to absorb B_{12} from your food, for instance, and smoking, aging, and stress all reduce your body's ability to digest and absorb folic acid. Look for a B-complex supplement that has 100 milligrams of B_1, 100 milligrams of B_2, 100 milligrams of niacin, 400 micrograms of folic acid, 100 micrograms of B_{12}, 100 micrograms of biotin, 100 milligrams of pantothenic acid, 50 milligrams of choline, and 100 milligrams of inositol. I take Vitamin Shoppe's B-Complex 100, which meets all those requirements.

Multivitamin. Think of your multivitamin as a nutrition insurance policy, especially on those days that you don't follow the Back-to-Life diet as well as you should. We all have those days. Even I have them. Look for a balanced multi that contains roughly 100 percent of the Daily Value for most nutrients (with the exception of calcium, which would not fit into such a small pill). I take TwinLab Daily One Caps without Iron.

Juice Plus. I learned about this product from Jamie, who learned about it from the world-famous and well-respected cardiologist Isadore Rosenfeld, M.D., with whom she cohosts *Sunday Housecall* on the FOX News Channel. It's a supplement that is packed with powdered fruit and vegetable juice. Although it's no substitute for the real thing, it's great to take as a little extra insurance, especially on those days when you might not Eat to Live as well as you'd like. You'll find it online at www.juiceplus.com.

Fish oil. Cold-water fish are rich in a type of polyunsaturated fat called omega-3 fatty acids. Many different studies show that consuming more of this type of fat—either from supplements or from food—both reduces risk of death from heart disease and slows the progression of heart disease. Fish oil may help stabilize your heart rhythm, lower levels of triglycerides (harmful fats in the bloodstream), keep your arteries clear of blockages, and reduce blood pressure. For instance, an Italian study of more than 11,000 heart attack survivors found that taking one daily capsule containing 850 combined milligrams of docosahexaenoic acid (DHA) and eicosapentaenoic acid (EPA) (the two main types of omega-3 fats in fish oil) cut their risk of death during the next three months by 40 percent. As an added bonus, it may also boost mood.

The Back to Life diet recommends that you eat fatty fish twice a week, but you'll benefit from a daily fish-oil supplement, too. Look for a supplement that supplies at least 2 grams of combined EPA and DHA. Only move up to 3 grams under a doctor's care, though, as fish oil thins the blood. Talk to your doctor before combining fish oil with aspirin or if you are taking a prescription blood thinner. Look for a flavored or purified brand to avoid a fishy aftertaste.

Resveratrol. This pigment produced by plants—particularly grapes and berries—wards off bacteria and other pathogens. Many experts think it is the magic ingredient that makes wine so healthy. As a supplement, resveratrol has been shown to increase the life span of a number of test creatures, including worms, yeast, and even fruit flies. It may improve health by acting as an antioxidant, scavenging the free radicals that lead to damaged arteries and cells. Take 250 milligrams daily.

Vitamin C. This vitamin is vital for the production of collagen, the protein material that forms our blood vessels. It also acts as a powerful antioxidant that neutralizes the free radicals that attack the lining of your arteries and lead to the damage that causes the body to build plaque in the first place. A University of California at Berkeley study found that vitamin C supplements lowered levels of C-reactive protein, a protein that indicates your level of heart-disease-causing inflammation.[7] A Harvard study found that vitamin C supplements reduced risk of heart attack by 28 percent in women.[8]

It's difficult to get enough vitamin C from your diet because this vitamin is so sensitive. Heat and oxygen destroy it, so cooking any vegetable

Larry Mart has a genetic disorder that prevents his body from adequately clearing cholesterol from his bloodstream. As a result, his cholesterol has been elevated since he was very young, perhaps since childhood. He suffered three heart attacks between ages twenty-nine and thirty-two, with the third one damaging a third of his heart muscle. After his first quintuple bypass at age thirty-three, doctors told him he had five years to live. Now another bypass and thirty years later, he's sixty-two and living life to the fullest. Here's how he does it.

————

After my third heart attack, I lost my business and had to apply for disability. My wife left me, too. All of my hopes and desires seemed to vanish. It took me about a year to realize that my life had forever changed. I realized that it would not do me any good to sit around and cry. I'd traveled the world while I was in the service. I'd seen how people in other countries lived. I realized I was still much better off than most of the world, even on my meager income.

So I figured out how to downsize and cut my expenses. I also surrounded myself with friends and family who cared about me, and I developed hobbies, such as photography and woodworking, that I love.

A few years later, I met the woman who would soon become my second wife. Together we built furniture, carved bowls, and made other woodworking creations.

I turned myself into a pretty decent cook, too, mostly in an effort to find a way to eat healthy low-fat, low-salt foods for less money. I've learned that the more food manufacturers take out of a given food, the more money they charge for the luxury of eating it! So to eat healthier, I bake my own bread and have made a project out of adapting high-fat recipes into low-fat ones. I've almost perfected low-fat pizza by baking my own crust and using low-fat meats and cheeses. I even make my own sausage with boneless, skinless chicken breast.

Over the years I've learned that our likes and dislikes of many foods are based on habit. You might try to eat something once and not like it. If you try eating it for about two weeks, it will grow on you. You can learn to like nearly anything.

Most of the time I'm religious about my diet, but every once in a while I go out and have a hot fudge sundae or a slice of pizza. It helps me keep my head on straight.

I've lived much longer than my doctors would have ever predicted, but I live with the certainty that, unless I get hit by a truck, I know how I am going to die. The only thing I don't know is when it's going to happen.

Heart disease has taught me to me thankful for the time I do have and to appreciate the small things in life. It has taught me to literally stop and smell the flowers. Every day I enjoy noticing things I've never noticed before. I've been walking down the same street for twenty years, but I might one day notice a new crack in the sidewalk or the color of the bark on a tree. I came close to dying, and now I am alive again. I have a second chance and I am going to make the best of it.

Larry's Unbeatable Advice: It's natural to feel sorry for yourself and think, "Why me?" and "What am I going to do?" after a major heart crisis. Eventually, however, you have to accept that life has changed and just start over. Figure out what you can still do and what you can no longer do and get on with it. It's the first day of the rest of your life.

will destroy most of its vitamin C content. Take a slow-release supplement that contains 1,000 milligrams of vitamin C a day.

Pycnogenol. Made from the bark of a pine tree, this antioxidant supplement may reduce blood clots, high blood pressure, and high blood cholesterol. A University of Arizona study of forty-eight people with type-2 diabetes found that it reduced heart disease risk. Half of the patients were able to normalize their blood pressure within twelve weeks by taking this supplement and others experienced a twelve-point drop in levels of LDL ("bad") cholesterol.[9] Take 200 milligrams daily.

Vitamin D. This is the new wonder vitamin, and many experts believe that up to half of us are deficient. Our bodies make it from sunlight, but most of us (especially anyone who lives north of Atlanta) don't get enough sunlight to make enough D during the late fall, winter, and early spring months.[10] Every cell in the body needs D to make countless reactions happen, and experts have now linked D deficiency with just about everything that can possibly ail us, including heart disease. A recent study done by Jefferson Medical College looked at government health statistics and nutritional surveys and determined that people with low blood levels of D were more likely to have heart disease than people with optimal blood levels.[11,12] Researchers now blame D deficiency for the increased incidence of heart attacks during the winter, when sunlight levels are lower. Ask your doctor to test your vitamin D levels during your next cholesterol screening. If you are deficient, take 1 to 2 IU every day, either as a stand-alone supplement or part of a multivitamin.

Getting Your Mind in the Healthy-Eating Game

You may need to confront any number of emotional demons as you systematically improve your diet. For example, like me, you may find yourself mired in an "it's not fair" cycle. Rather than actually doing something about the way you eat, you continually remind yourself that it's not fair that you have to eat differently than people who don't have heart disease. Well, you know what would be really unfair? If your bad eating habits continually worsened your disease.

You may also find that you are stuck in the past, blaming circumstances that are beyond your control rather than doing what you can to get healthy now. For example, at first I blamed my blockages on my genetics and on the fact that during my teenage years and through my surgical residency I lived on fast food and pizza. I knew that I could do better, and eventually I did.

Finally, you may find yourself mired in denial, and this denial is something that you will find you have to continually fight. You might find yourself saying things like, "I had bypass surgery. It doesn't matter what I eat. I'm fixed."

Yes, you are fixed for now, but if you don't change your eating habits, you won't be fixed for long. Don't you want to live to experience your kids and grandkids? Do you want to travel to places you've never been? Then Eat to Live. It's the best insurance policy there is for a long, healthy life.

❋   **BACK TO LIFE R$_x$**   ❋

- Water + Vegetables + Fruit + Lean protein (poultry, fish, eggs) + culinary joy (a little wine, a little chocolate, a little olive oil) = Eating to Live
- Eat to live as often as possible so you can live a long, healthy life
- Live to eat every once in a while so you can live a long, happy life

---

9

Step 7:
Arm Yourself
for Career Issues

THE FIRST TIME I WALKED BACK INTO THE HOSPITAL WHERE I WORKED, it had been nearly two months since my operation. My mind was filled with questions: "Who am I going to be? What am I going to be able to do? Will I ever be the same?"

Before I went back, I'd imagined I would feel like a Purple Heart veteran coming back from a war. Here I was, a man who had faced his mortality. I'd lived through having my chest bone sawed open. I wanted my colleagues to admire me for that.

Deep down, however, I was nervous. I worried that my coworkers and patients would see my thin body (I still had not regained all my weight) and think, "Is he still sick? Can he really handle this?" I felt as if I was the new kid in school, the one whose mom dressed him in the dorky outfit. My dorky outfit was a suit that didn't fit.

I also knew that I didn't have the stamina that I'd once had. I asked for a couch to be sent to my office so I could rest during the day, as needed. I arranged to have the administrative secretary hold my calls for twenty minutes once a day so I could relax and recharge. I knew I needed to do this, but I worried, "Will my colleagues see it as a sign of weakness?" I wasn't sure whether I should be open about my limitations or whether I should hide them instead.

I worried about so many things. Did I have the stamina needed to stand in the OR for as many hours as it took to finish a complicated surgery? What if something went wrong and a surgery took more time than I could handle? I arranged to make sure another senior surgeon was always in the OR with me, just in case I felt fatigued and needed someone to take over.

And then there were the comments and questions from physicians and staff. Few people knew how to react. Some stared at me and said nothing. Others were overly helpful. For instance, I used to sit outside the OR just after a surgery, waiting for the staff to turn the room over. Periodically someone on staff would see me sitting there and say, "Are you tired? You look tired. Maybe you should lie down and rest." They meant well, but such comments made me feel weak.

What I wasn't prepared for at all was the backbiting and the jockeying among physicians who wanted my job and who would do nearly anything they could to use my illness against me.

For instance, I vividly remember attending a meeting at work during my initial months back. In the room were some of the more distinguished members of the hospital community, people who knew about diseases and how they progressed, people who *knew better.*

We had gathered to talk about the hospital's financial situation. At that time, St. Vincent's was not doing well. The CEO had been removed, and a consulting company had been hired to turn things around. We all knew that heads were about to roll. I made a few comments about what I thought was needed to save the hospital. A colleague in the room said, "Why are you listening to him? He's impaired. He doesn't really know what he is saying. He had a heart attack." Heart attack told everyone that heart muscle was damaged. This was not the case. I caught the angina before any heart muscle died.

I was floored. I could not believe it. I thought, "Heart attack? I didn't have a heart attack! And even if I had, I'm thinking just fine, thank you very much!" Yet behind that tough exterior the comment chipped away at my confidence, and questions pervaded my thinking. *Am I thinking clearly? Am I compromised? Am I impaired? Can I do this job? Am I the man, the surgeon, the scientist, and the administrator I used to be?* I should have said, "Excuse me?" I should have defended myself. Instead I just went along with it, as if it were all some funny joke.

A few months later during the winter, I walked into a different meeting. I'd just come into the hospital from the outside. I was dressed in a warm coat, hat, and earmuffs. After the meeting, a coworker pulled me aside and said, "You cannot come into a conference room while wearing a hat and a coat. You look sick and weak. You've got to stop doing this."

I realized that he was telling me this not to reprimand me, but rather as a way of looking out for me. He was warning me that others would try to use my illness against me, but the words still stung. I felt awful.

I could see how this was going to go. Whenever I made the slightest mistake, whenever I accidentally said right instead of left, whenever I

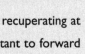

JAMIE'S ADVICE FOR CAREGIVERS

Marc's transition back to work started while he was recuperating at home. A few weeks into his recovery, I asked his assistant to forward some of his mail to the house. I gave her very specific instructions, too, asking her to sort the mail into three categories:

1. Anything that would make him smile or laugh: Send it right away.
2. Anything she could take care of without his help: Don't send it. Handle it in the office.
3. Anything pressing that he either needed to see or sign: Send it, but only two or three of such important matters at a time.

A couple weeks later, I suggested he invite some people from the office over for a meeting. His research fellows and assistant came and they all sat around the table and brainstormed topics. I supplied lunch and made the atmosphere as festive as possible, but I made sure Marc ate before the meeting so he wouldn't feel self-conscious. I also made sure that no medical apparatus—heating pads, pills, cushions—were visible. That way Marc didn't have to worry about his research fellows noticing how much or how little he ate or how sick he looked. Yes, it was difficult for him, but not as difficult as it would have been to go straight from home to office life with no in-between. This allowed him to ease his way back into things.

I helped him plan his first day back at the office, too. I made sure he did not schedule back-to-back surgeries. We even wrote out his to-do list at home, so he had plenty of time to think about what he could handle and what he couldn't.

The day before he went back, I took him to the barbershop and splurged for a cut and shave. It was just a little extra pampering that would allow him to feel as pulled together as possible.

Then on the first day, I made sure he had money in his wallet, the right pills in his pill dispenser, the phone number for his doctor, and snacks to eat throughout the day. I tried to take care of such small details so he could start his first day back feeling as relaxed as possible. I also scheduled an appointment with his doctor a few days before so he would feel as confident as possible about his ability to work.

I drove him to work that day, too. He could have driven himself, of course. He'd been driving for a while at that point. Still, this allowed me to kiss him and wish him a good day. I'm sure it was also reassuring for him to know that he could call me to pick him up at any time.

walked down the wrong hallway—whenever I made any number of very normal mistakes that most people make every day and either laugh off or don't think about at all—a colleague would notice and blame it on my heart disease. At one time someone said, "He's not what he once was. See? He's compromised."

I again feel on top of my game—as a surgeon, as an administrator, and as a researcher. I have the respect now of my staff, colleagues, and patients. I not only enjoy my work, but also look forward to it. What I do for a living is certainly challenging, but it's the kind of challenging that gets me out of bed in the morning. No matter what your current work situation, you can get back on top of your game, too. If I did it, so can you.

Hopefully, your back-to-work experience will go nothing like mine! Ideally, you'll return to a workplace where empathetic coworkers are there for you to lean on and where no one tries to use your limitations against you. If your workplace is similar to mine, however, the advice throughout this chapter will help you swim with the sharks without losing a limb!

Before You Go Back

Take off as much time as you can. Look into filing for disability, but do it through a lawyer or insurance agent and not through your place of employment, if possible. You don't need people in the office talking about how you are "disabled." Believe me.

If you don't qualify for your disability coverage, see how many sick and vacation days you can use, and consider taking some unpaid leave as well. Take as long as you can. If you think you look tired and weak, then it's probably too early to return to work. You want to look as rested and refreshed as possible. More important, you want to feel that way, too.

See your doctor before you go back. Prepare a list of questions, asking what you are ready for, and what you aren't. Can you work outside in cold weather? Can you work outside in hot weather? Can you lift heavy objects? What about taking the stairs? What can you expect in terms of stamina and attention span? How many hours will you be able to work productively before you will need a break? How much caffeine can you safely drink if you need a little pick-me-up? How long will you be able to sit at a computer before you feel fatigued and need to rest? How often will you need pain medicine, and should your dose change once you return to working life? What medicines should you make sure you always have with you? Run through what usually happens during a typical day at your office so your doctor can help you plan your initial days back. That way you can go back to work knowing what you can handle, and what you can't.

Finally, prepare your one-liners. Coworkers are going to ask you the same questions over and over again. Know how you will answer certain questions before you ever step foot in the office door. Practice saying, "I'm great. I'm fine!" Be prepared to answer, "No! I feel great," when people ask you if you are tired. Be prepared to say, "Work is great," when people ask you about your first day. Think of short, upbeat, positive answers, and use the same ones over and over again. This will reduce the stress and anxiety of the persistent questioning from your coworkers.

Your First Day

Use this advice to ease your transition back to working life.

Make your first day a half day. And don't schedule anything very pressing. Just use it to get used to the day-to-day office happenings, to get caught up on e-mail, to return phone calls, and to get caught up with your coworkers. Only schedule tasks for yourself that you know without a doubt you can accomplish. You want to inspire courage in yourself, and you want your coworkers to see you being capable and effective.

Wear long underwear. If you've lost a lot of weight, you'll probably feel colder than usual at work, so dress in layers. If you have a private office, consider bringing in a small space heater.

Wear comfortable clothing. You want to look as professional as possible, of course, but don't dress up so much that you feel weighed down by your clothes. For instance, it's okay not to wear a tie at first, especially if your incision is still tender.

Get to work in the least stressful way possible. You don't need to battle traffic on your first day. See if someone can drop you off and pick you up.

Find an inconspicuous way to store and take your meds. That way you won't have to worry about people seeing all those medicine bottles and wondering if you are still sick. Put them in a medicine dispenser that you carry with you. Don't discuss your meds with anyone at work. I learned this the hard way. Some of my colleagues judged me by the medications I was taking.

Clean up your office. On my first day back, when I opened my desk drawer, I found a number of bottles of Excedrin, Tums, and other reminders of my stressful workload. Get rid of such reminders. You are no longer a stressed-out workaholic who needs to live on caffeine, sugar, and painkillers.

Job Stress and Your Heart

Before my bypass, the stress I internalized from my job, family responsibilities, and the world around me almost killed me—literally.

The year leading up to my bypass was particularly stressful. It started on September 11, 2001, when terrorists attacked the World Trade Center and the towers collapsed. This tragedy affected me greatly as a New Yorker. As Chief of Surgery at St. Vincent's Hospital, it touched me even more deeply. St. Vincent's served as the main triage hospital to treat the victims, and I supervised triage that day. On an even deeper level, my wife went to Ground Zero to report the story. She was there when the towers fell, and I was unable to communicate with her for hours. I spent a great deal of the day worried about her well-being. I had the double sadness of witnessing the event and worrying about losing the woman I loved so deeply. I had many sleepless nights following that day.

Then in March 2002 a close friend and trusted colleague, Dr. Dennis Tyras, was killed in a car accident. He was driving to meet me for an early-morning meeting when a steel rod fell off a truck traveling in the opposite direction, boomeranged, and hit his car, decapitating him. The hospital administration asked me to break the tragic news to his wife. That definitely was another hit, and a major stressor for my heart.

The same month, my mother fainted in the lobby of her apartment house and was hospitalized. While she was recovering, I came home from work feeling dead tired, and then spent three or four hours with her in the hospital. This was the beginning of several health scares and ministrokes for her. Seeing her health fail emphasized my own mortality, and I became more frazzled as a result.

Two months later, my stepson Greg informed his mother and me that he planned to move to Kentucky to be near his biological father. I had raised him since he was two, and the news stung deeply. I'd thrown myself 100 percent into raising him with Jamie. During his time away, we were all mired in conflict, which weighed heavily on me.

Then, in June, Jamie learned she had been passed over for a promotion she was sure she would get. She had put in countless hours freelancing in this position, even risked her life reporting 9/11, only to be passed over.

Sometimes I think back on the events of that year and I think, "No wonder I needed a bypass!" Stress is bad for every cell in your body, and it has been linked with practically every disease you can name, including heart disease. Indeed, some researchers believe chronic stress is as bad for your health as smoking.[1]

When you are under stress, your nervous system responds by releasing stress hormones including adrenaline and cortisol. These hormones cause your heart to beat faster, muscles to tighten, blood pressure to rise, and so on. They ready your body to flee or fight.

But in most work situations, you do neither. Your emergency stress-response system is on, and it stays on because you do nothing to reduce the stress. If you've ever owned a pet, then you know that most animals have natural coping strategies for stress. When you yell at your dog for eating from the kitchen garbage can, you've probably noticed that he soon responds with a wild attack—racing around the house like a maniac. He's unloading the stress from his system in a healthy way.

Most humans, however, don't do this. We stew in stress instead, so the stress hormones remain elevated. This sets off a series of ill effects: elevating blood pressure, suppressing the immune system, and increasing blood sugar chronically, for instance. Stress may slow your recovery. It might even interfere with medications you're taking.

Consider:

- Research on heart attack survivors determined that chronic work strain doubles the odds of experiencing a second heart attack over ten years.[2]
- A ten-year-long Danish study of 2,465 bus drivers (an occupation that comes with a high risk for developing heart disease) determined that drivers who had routes in highly trafficked areas (and therefore were more likely to be stressed) had higher rates of heart disease.[3]

Studies have also linked chronic stress with an increased risk of heart attack, stroke, arrhythmia, blood clots, and hardening of the arteries.[4,5,6,7]

None of this was good news for me, as my job was and still is stressful on a day-to-day basis. During a typical fifteen- to seventeen-hour day, I split my time between office work, clinic, the operating room, teaching, training, research, caregiving, and administrating. I also spent a great deal of time with my patients, helping many of them deal with their eventual deaths. After years of caring for certain patients, it is a great personal loss to let any of them go.

Because I worked as an administrator, I was also one of the chief complaint receptacles for the physicians on staff. I listened to their grievances about their income, the conditions of the operating rooms, the ways the head nurses manage the floors, and even how well the urinals work in the bathrooms. I've heard it all. Think *Grey's Anatomy* meets *The Apprentice* and you'll get an idea of some of the stress I faced every day. But soon it was the stress my colleagues caused me that took its toll. I began to feel scrutinized all the time, and it caused me tremendous anxiety.

In one incident from that period of time, a colleague even questioned my fitness as a surgeon. I had repaired a ventral hernia on a patient. These types of hernias are pesky, and they tend to recur roughly 40 percent of the time. The patient had been older, overweight, and on medication, all of which tend to increase the recurrence rate. And I was doing a follow-up surgery on this patient as it was. The initial surgery, one I did not do, had failed, and the hernia had come back.

Which is exactly what happened about three months after I repaired it. The patient was back, yet again, for yet another hernia repair.

This was the type of thing that was normal. At a routine conference where we talk about how we complete surgeries, what complications may have hindered the success, and anything that we might do differently in the future to prevent such complications, this colleague took it upon himself to highlight this surgery as an example of my inability to operate.

Me? The person who was so careful in the OR?

I was so stunned that I did not know how to react.

I ended up feeling paranoid about everyone and everything because he and one other physician seemed to be picking apart my every move. If I didn't drink coffee at a meeting, I worried someone would whisper behind my back, "He doesn't drink coffee. That must be because it's bad for his heart!" If I didn't eat a certain food, I worried someone would say, "Look, he has no appetite. He must still be really sick."

I would love to tell you that I made the necessary career changes quickly and easily. That would be a lie. Ultimately, I was asked to step down. I was told that my coworkers no longer held me in the same regard as when I was chairman.

I was scared. My entire world turned upside down. My research and a part-time position I held at another hospital would net me a third of my usual salary. Would I be able to continue to pay our mortgage? Would I be able to provide for my family? It seemed as if my worst fears were coming true. I lay in bed awake many nights, trying to figure out how to salvage my career. In fact, I was again suffering some of the same thoughts that I went through after undergoing open-heart surgery.

My wife reminded me that my position was what I did; it was not who I was. Looking back on it, however, I now realize it was one of the best things that could ever have happened for my health. Of course, I miss my former residents and all my private-practice patients whom the hospital retained, but I was able to turn my hardship into an opportunity.

I took that part-time position at another hospital and eventually turned it into a full-time job. I now work closer to home with people whom I trained and trust. At Metropolitan Hospital, I care for and operate on the

I don't know about your husband, but mine is one of those men who thrives on work. I suppose you could call him a workaholic. Before his bypass, Marc worked fifteen-hour days. Then the moment he walked in the front door, the phone started ringing. It was always some doctor or another coworker who wanted to discuss one problem or another with him.

He felt as if he had to be the first physician in the hospital doors and the last one out. He thought he had to complete the most surgeries. He thought he had to do every duty—including night call—that other physicians handled, even though he was an administrator. He tried to be the perfect doctor.

I knew Marc was the type of man who would want to put on a suit and go right back to those fifteen-hour days. I also knew that wasn't good for his health. I saw him worrying about work. I watched him growing more and more tense and stressed-out. Not long after he lost his job, I blew my stack and I let him have it. Loudly and in rapid-fire speech, without giving him a moment to say the word "but," I said, "Let me just tell you this. Your job is what you do. It is not who you are. Your job is what pays for your food and your clothes and your lifestyle. It facilitates your life, but it is not your life. You are Marc Wallack. You have a caring heart. You are a wonderful father and the best husband around. But you are not your job. Your job is just a job. It is not who you are. You need to remind yourself that over and over and over again."

That speech completely changed him. He realized that he might not have control over his heart, but he did have control over his job and the stress that he internalized because of it. To help reduce his stress

> load, he stopped taking business calls from complaining colleagues at night. When people suggested business meetings over dinner, he suggested a 7 a.m. breakfast meeting at his office. He stopped enabling the colleagues who disabled him. Now the sentences "Your job is what you do. It's not who you are" have become two of his favorites.

underserved in the clinic. I've learned some Spanish to communicate better with my Spanish-speaking patients, and to some extent I'm still able to teach the residents and medical students I care so much about.

Do You Need a Career Change?

For various reasons, you may not be able to go back to your old job. Your health may not allow it or your coworkers or supervisors may not treat you with enough compassion.

How do you know if your job is too stressful? You are under too much job stress if you have:

- Chronic headaches or muscle tension
- Chronic stomach problems
- Loss of sex drive
- Chronic fatigue
- Insomnia
- Chronic anxiety or depression

If you are miserable in your job, you must realize that you are not stuck. You are in control. You have three choices:

Make the time your spouse arrives home from work a special time for the two of you. Encourage your spouse to rest for a while once he or she walks in the door. Then ask him or her about the day's events. Be prepared to hold a hand and listen for a long while. Marc, for instance, came home nearly every day with stories about someone looking at him the wrong way or saying something stupid.

Also, notice how your spouse looks at the end of the workday. If, after a few weeks, he comes home looking worse and worse, it may be time for a job change. To figure out whether his job is truly toxic or whether he just feels temporarily overwhelmed due to all that is involved with his recovery, ask him these questions:

1. Are you feeling physically and emotionally fatigued because you are sad or because you truly can no longer handle your job?

2. Could your medication be making you feel this way? Should we talk to your doctor about adjusting your medicines?

3. Is there someone at work who can take on some of your job responsibilities, at least temporarily, until you are feeling back to your old self again? But this person must be completely trustworthy and understanding. If not, the answer is no.

4. Can we ask your HR department to accommodate you so your job can be a perfect fit until you feel perfect?

1. You can stay in this job and try to improve it from within, by asking for a different position or work responsibilities. Under the Americans with Disabilities Act, you may be eligible for accommodations, al-

though asking for these accommodations increases your risk of being viewed and treated as "sick."

2. You can do nothing and stay miserable until someone else decides to take action.

3. You can look for a new job.

I made choice number 2. Don't make that choice! It's better to be in control of your own destiny than to wait and allow others to control it for you. Consider making changes in your current job or finding a new job, but don't give up on working. I've counseled many survivors who decide not to work at all. Don't consider this as an option if you don't have to, especially if you believe that your career defined you before your health crisis. You may not go back to your original job, but you do need to find something that improves your confidence and self-worth.

How to Improve Your Current Situation

According to studies about the health impacts of job strain, there are three important variables to keep in mind:[8]

1. The psychological demand of your day-to-day work.

2. How in control you feel at work. In other words, do you choose your projects and work responsibilities, or do they choose you?

3. Your level of support, from either coworkers, friends, or your loved ones.

If the psychological demands of the job are high and the level of control and support are low, you've got a recipe brewing for worsening your heart disease. Now here's the thing: Many people focus on changing the first variable—the psychological demands of the job. Yet of the three variables, this may actually be the least important when it comes to job strain and your health.

Many self-employed business owners, for instance, face tough psychological demands, yet most report they are more content than ever. Why? They are completely in control of their lives. It isn't inherently bad for your health to work in a high-stress profession such as teaching, law enforcement, or medicine. What's bad for your health is the sensation that your job is out of your control and that no one cares. This is critical for you to understand. I wish I'd understood it at the time I needed to most. My job was out of my control, but I was not smart enough to move on.

Here are some ways to increase your sense of control as you decrease your level of work stress.

Get moving. The healthier and stronger you are physically, the better able you will be to cope with stress. Exercise lifts your mood, reduces anxiety, increases energy, and sharpens your focus. It also makes you much more resilient. If you haven't already started a cardiac rehabilitation program, start one now. In the next chapter, I'll outline some specific ways to get in shape. For now, know that doing so is one of the best ways to prove to your coworkers that you are healthy. I quite often leave work and go for a quick walk outside, especially during those moments of the day when I feel stressed and need to clear my head.

During my initial months back to work, I left work three times a week at 1 p.m. so I could work out at a gym for my cardiac rehab. I'd get back to work around 3:30 and I'd make up the lost time by working late. That I was so committed to my recovering and my health drove my coworkers crazy, especially the surgeons who thought they could do better. I looked at it this way: I'd rather they be irritated with me and I be alive than they be happy and I be dead. My life became much more important than my job.

Telecommute. Initially look into working some of your time at home. This will save you the stress of commuting and dealing with difficult co-workers. You can use all sorts of technology these days to stay in touch with the office without actually being in the office. You can attend meetings with teleconferencing or Skype. You can share documents through Google docs, and you can instant message as needed.

Just say no. Delegate whenever possible. If you are self-employed, look into using a part-time or virtual assistant (a secretary whom you hire through the Internet). Outsource other tasks: technical help, cleaning, accounting . . . anything and everything that makes sense. Go easy on yourself. This is your life.

If you work for a company, use whatever existing support staff you can. That's what they are there for. If they don't back you up or just don't get it, then they are not there for you. Perhaps they are the ones who should lose their jobs!

Mellanie True Hills was a successful consultant who worked for companies such as JCPenney, Dell, and Cisco Systems to develop corporate Internet and Intranet sites and strategies. During a business trip, she experienced shortness of breath and pain in her left shoulder. While doctors were testing and treating her, she was returning customer phone calls, thinking about an upcoming tax deadline, and asking her husband to run home to get her laptop. The doctors did an emergency angioplasty, placing a stent inside one artery to prop it open. She was fifty-one at the time.

———

Initially I wondered, "What would have happened had I not made it?" Soon, however, I turned that around 180 degrees and said to myself, "Now I have a chance to make sure I will make it. What kinds of changes do I need to make? What does this mean for me? How do I embrace this and use it to determine what I should be doing next?"

To reduce my level of stress, I had to keep reminding myself that my health is my most important priority, that if I am not taking care of myself, I will not be here to take care of others. I had to constantly remind myself that putting my health first is not selfish. That was a big mind-set shift.

Once I made that shift, though, it was easier for me to say no to certain commitments. It was easier for me to make the choice to walk rather than work as I waited for a flight. It was easier for me to take time off, too. I even took a trip with my family across the country in our motor home—with little e-mail or cell phone access!

Once I got my healthy habits under control, I began to look into giving back—into using what I learned from this disease to help others.

I began volunteering for the American Heart Association and speaking about women and heart disease in an effort to help other women avoid what I'd been through. I went on to found the American Foundation for Women's Health, a nonprofit organization dedicated to educating women about health issues. I've turned what could have been a life-ending illness into my life's work.

Just seven months later, though, I was diagnosed with atrial fibrillation. I'd never heard of it. I learned there was a problem with my heart's electrical system that caused it to beat erratically. I was put on medication to treat it.

Despite the medication, I began to have episodes when it felt as if my heart was racing or skipping beats. I would get so dizzy and light-headed that I thought I would pass out. I never knew when an episode would strike, so I was always afraid.

I eventually decided to undergo minimally invasive surgery on the nerves and tissues around my heart to block the electrical signals that were disrupting my heart. I have no regrets. I can now fly again and travel by myself. I eventually decided to use this experience to help others, so I created StopAfib.org, a nonprofit online community of support and information for afib patients. I have now been afib-free for three years, and I am thankful every day that I have my life back. Every day I feel blessed to be here.

Mellanie's Unbeatable Advice: Many women feel selfish when they put themselves first. They nurture others and take care of everyone else, but run out of time to take care of themselves. Putting yourself first isn't selfish. Not doing so is selfish. If you don't care for yourself and your health, you won't be here to care for others.

Solve problems with creativity and assertiveness. Ask people to come to your office for a meeting during those initial days and weeks back at the office, for instance, so you don't have to walk farther than you feel able to. If you work in sales and worry that your clients won't trust you because you still look sick, deal with them over the phone or by using Skype through your computer.

Balance your schedule. You need a balance among work, family, and life. It's important to have a social life. It's important to have some downtime. Do you really need to take papers home with you at night? Do you really need to answer the phone when your coworkers call you at home, especially on the weekends?

Just say, "Have fun!" Jamie's brother Jonathan Colby, a retired judge and attorney, gave us this tip, and we've both been grateful, because it really works. You know those buttons they sell at Staples that say "Easy"? One day, he told us to try what he'd done for years. Imagine an invisible button, just like that, on your desk, only instead of "easy" it says, "Have fun!" Jamie and I now have our own little invisible buttons on our desks, and whenever we feel a little overwhelmed with work life, we bang on those buttons and feel instantly better. Trust us. It works.

Create an office oasis. Play classical or some other type of relaxing music, using headphones if needed. Or bring in a sound machine or water garden and anything else you find soothing. Make the appearance, sounds, and smells of your office as soothing as possible. This is extremely important if you had any sort of chest pain while you were at work. Redecorate your office as much as possible, so it doesn't remind you of heart disease. Use aromatherapy. In the beginning, when I returned to work, I burned incense or a candle, using scents that I found pleasing and relaxing. I also bought a miniature waterfall for my desk.

Allow your to-do list to go undone. Keep a to-do list if it helps you stay on track, but don't become a slave to it. Don't schedule appointments back-to-back. Create breathing room in your day. Drop tasks that are not absolutely necessary.

Split up your work tasks into "musts" and "it would be nice." If you can't get something done on the "would be nice" list, leave it for the next workday. I know this is easier said than done, but face it—if your life ends because of stress over your to-do list, does it really matter what's left on that list?

Breathe deeply. Whenever I notice my heart beginning to race, I breathe deeply. Usually in four to five deep breaths, I feel calmer and more productive. Inhale into your abdomen, so it expands with air. Then your rib cage and finally your chest will expand, too. Then let go slowly and repeat four or five times.

Play music. Listen to calming music in the car, at work (through headphones, if needed), and wherever else you tend to feel stressed. I've found music particularly helpful. I still keep a CD player and a small desktop fountain on my desk.

Take a break. I still work long days, but I don't put in all the hours back-to-back. I encourage you to take one to two fifteen-minute breaks a day. Listen to your body. When you feel tired, don't fight it. Find a place to lie down and rest or go for a slow walk, taking slow deep breaths. This will help clear your mind and allow your body to recover.

Create a support posse. Build a supportive community of people. These may be people who you might not have previously gotten to know. In my case, the kindest and most compassionate coworkers had nothing to do with my day-to-day job. They were the cleaning and security staff. Every day they smiled my way, and those smiles got me through a lot.

Limit coffee. It's okay to have a little caffeine—about a half-cup of coffee—but know that it will make your heart rate accelerate. Also, if you are the typical type-A personality (like me), then be careful not to slip into those old type-A habits of using caffeine to fuel a super-stressful day.

Eat regularly. Remember those small frequent meals we talked about in Chapter 8? Keep that up after you return to work. Having five meals and snacks a day—rather than just two or three—will keep your blood sugar stable. You'll have more energy and be better able to handle stress. To make sure you eat regularly, stash convenient snacks in your office, such as Ensure shakes. I purchased a very small refrigerator for under my desk. It holds about six Ensures and water.

Stop trying to be perfect. You put undue stress on yourself by trying to do everything perfectly. You are only human—and so is everyone else!

See if you can change your job description. Talk with your supervisor about tailoring your job to your skills and energy level or consider a lateral transfer to a less stressful position. Rehearse this discussion ahead of time with a therapist, spouse, or close friend (not someone from your workplace).

Report abuse to Human Resources. Federal laws protect people with disabilities. Your company cannot legally discriminate against you because you have heart disease or are recovering from heart surgery. If someone is gunning for your job, walk into Human Resources with a note from your doctor requesting the accommodations you need. Do you need a ten-minute nap once a day? Take one, stay ten minutes later at night, and get your doctor to put it in writing. It's a lot harder for a company to fire you once you've gone public.

And continually remind yourself: Your job is what you do. It's not who

❖ THE UNBEATABLES ❖

Yvonne Payne was diagnosed with a heart rhythm disorder when she was a teenager. She's lived her adult life with one type of defibrillator or another implanted in her chest. During her most recent surgery to implant yet another device, doctors experienced difficulty and almost lost her, shocking her heart ten times to bring her back. It took her four months to get back on her feet, and she may eventually need a transplant. Here's how she reclaimed her life.

————

When I woke from surgery and saw my entire family gathered around me, I knew something had gone wrong. I knew they wouldn't all be there if it hadn't. But I was in denial. People kept trying to tell me what had happened, but I blocked it all out. I did not want to hear it. I would not let them explain it to me.

I was in so much emotional and physical pain, too. When they shock your heart like that, it feels like someone has hit you with a baseball bat, over and over and over. I just gave up. I really didn't care if I died. I just wanted it to be over. It was hard just to talk to other people because, although they were supportive, I felt alone. I didn't feel as if they could ever comprehend what I was going through. I thought I was going to die.

But my husband kept printing out information about my heart condition and possible treatments for what was wrong. He kept giving me positive feedback, and that helped a lot. I also did a lot of praying.

Over time, as I healed and got stronger, I was able to face the situation and start fighting.

Now, four months later, I can finally go up and down steps and walk on a treadmill. I know I am getting better. I still get panicky and anxious, especially when I'm getting a bad heart rhythm. I have great days when my heart beats normally all day. Then I have bad days when I have to sit down and wait until a bad rhythm passes. Because of this, doctors tell me that, in two to three years, I may need a transplant. I could obsess about that and allow it to freak me out, or I could focus on the present and deal with the future when the future comes.

Now I want to live. I want to be able to be around for my family and friends. I want to be able to do things. My life isn't finished. I have not fulfilled my purpose yet. I want to find a way to use what has happened to me as a way to help and give to others. To me the act of giving makes me feel wonderful. It gives me the chills. God blessed me so I can bless others, and that is what gives me the meaning I need to keep trying.

Yvonne's Unbeatable Advice: Don't give up. You have a chance, a second chance to live again. Take care of yourself. Eat right and exercise. Fight. This is a battle that you have to fight, and it will be very, very rough. You have to hang in there. I'm still going through a lot myself. I'm still fighting, and it's not easy, but I'm not going to give up, and you shouldn't either.

you are. I learned this from Jamie and now I believe it. Avoid negative coworkers, and congratulate yourself about small accomplishments, even if no one else does.

When It's Time to Move On

You may find, as I did, that you simply cannot continue to work in the same environment you did before your heart disease diagnosis. If you decide to move on, think about the following:

Your interests. What do you love? Is there something you've always wanted to do but have been too scared to try? Is there something that you didn't do because you thought you wouldn't make enough money or garner enough status by doing it? Think about the former addicts who become counselors, the breast cancer survivors who become health advocates, the successful dieters who become fitness instructors. Perhaps this journey has taught you something that you can learn from and pass on to others.

Your options. What career options match your interests?

Once you settle on a few ideas, research what you need to have in place in order to make a career jump. Do you need special training? Do you need to go back to school? Could you learn some skills through an apprenticeship? Can you learn the ropes as a volunteer, intern, or part-timer?

If needed, pick a short-term job just to pay the bills—something that you can handle that's not too stressful—as well as a long-term dream job that you slowly work toward. Before you ever think about leaving one job, make sure you have made contacts and have lined up financial support. No matter what, though, never give up. Just as there is a next chapter after a heart trauma, there is a next chapter for your career. You can remake yourself and your career and emerge more confident, happy, and calm.

- Delegate tasks to others. You are only human.
- Hit the "Have fun!" button, as needed.
- Create an office oasis.
- Fill out that "I accomplished" list daily.
- Take breathing and walking breaks, as needed.

10

Step 8:
Train for a Huge
Physical Challenge

I REALIZED I NEEDED TO RUN A MARATHON AFTER WATCHING A PAR-ticular episode of *The Sopranos,* the HBO drama about Mafia life. In it Mob boss Tony Soprano is recovering from a near-fatal gunshot wound. He's lost respect from his colleagues, most of whom seem to be jockeying to take his place. To protect himself, he has a huge bodyguard with him at all times.

One day, in front of "the boys," he berates his bodyguard for bringing him the wrong beer from the refrigerator. It was, in Tony's opinion, not cold enough. Tony's wounds are still fresh. His face is still pale. He looks like death warmed over, but he beats this guy—this huge, meaty, strong guy—to a pulp, showing his colleagues once and for all that he is indestructible and undefeatable. Then he goes to the bathroom and throws up.

I loved that episode because I completely understood Tony's situation. I was going through similar problems at work, with colleagues who assumed I was weak and damaged and who wanted to take me out. As I watched Tony Soprano prove his virility by taking on the biggest, baddest challenge he could—the bodyguard—I knew I needed to do the same.

Tony's bodyguard was my marathon.

Your bodyguard might not be a marathon, but it will be something physical. To fully recover mentally and physically from heart disease, you need to take on that one thing you most fear. Only then will you prove to yourself and others that you are back and better than ever.

Why We All Need a Challenge

After a major health catastrophe, there's nothing like a physical challenge to prove to yourself that you really are alive. There's nothing like physical exhaustion to blast away stress, take your mind off your troubles, and lift your mood. There's nothing like pushing yourself physically to prove to yourself that you really are okay, even if that means walking faster and faster in a mall all year round.

Challenge allows us to overcome our fears, doubts, and frustrations.

I recommend you challenge yourself in a way that you may have never challenged yourself before. Don't worry. I'm not going to make you run a marathon. I won't even force you to run a single step. I will, however, encourage you to get physically fit and then, once you do so, challenge yourself by signing up for something scary—it could be a walkathon, a charity bike ride, or an endurance swim. You get to pick the challenge. I'll help walk you through the process.

Step 1: Get in Shape

You can't challenge yourself physically until you feel physically well, so your first step involves getting in shape. Improve your fitness so you can do the minimum amount of exercise recommended by the American Heart Association and other heart-disease experts.

Regular exercise is crucial for getting and staying healthy. It reduces your risk of heart disease by lowering blood pressure, triglycerides, cholesterol, and body fat, and improving circulation and blood sugar control.[1,2] Specifically, it helps boost levels of the good HDL cholesterol. Low levels of HDL (less than 40 mg/dL for men and less than 50 mg/dL for women) have been linked to a higher risk of heart disease. Physical activity can significantly increase HDL cholesterol levels and thus reduce your risk.[3]

As a result, regular exercise lengthens your life and reduces your risk of a heart attack. The results of many, many studies show that people who start regular physical activity after having a heart attack have better rates of survival and better quality of life.

As a side benefit, exercise also helps boost mood and reduce stress. It can help you stick to other healthy habits such as heart-healthy eating. Many smokers find that regular exercise helps them kick the habit, too.

Exercise also strengthens your muscles so you can stay strong as you age. It prevents bone loss, lowers your risk for certain cancers, boosts energy, improves sleep, and generally makes you feel good. Because you feel good, you'll become more effective at just about everything you do.

The opposite—sitting still—is one of the most preventable causes of death.

The problem with exercise is this: Its benefits cannot be turned into a handy little pill and marketed in a bottle. Seriously, if all the benefits of regular exercise could be bottled, it would surely become one of the most expensive and highly sought-after pills on the market! Alas, the only way to reap these benefits of exercise is by living this mantra: "Move more, sit less."

Marc's Back-to-Life Exercise Plan

I recommend three types of exercise.[4]

Cardiovascular exercise (cardio). This speeds your heart rate. It includes brisk walking, jogging, swimming, cycling, dancing, skating, and much more.

Dose: At least thirty minutes every day of purposeful movement such as power walking or lifestyle movement—taking the stairs instead of the elevator, for example. See How to Do Cardio on pages 212 to 216 for guidance.

Strength training. This does just as it says: It strengthens your muscles and bones. This is critically important, because stronger muscles do much more than make your groceries easier to lug from the car to the house. Muscle is active body tissue, with busy little cells that need a robust calorie supply in order to function. As a result, stronger muscles help your body more efficiently process blood sugar and fat, helping normalize levels of blood cholesterol, triglycerides, and blood sugar.

A West Virginia University study of thousands of people determined that strength training helped lower total cholesterol, boost the good HDL cholesterol, lower the bad LDL cholesterol, and drop triglycerides. It also helps improve blood-sugar control and drops blood pressure.

Consult your doctor if you notice any of the following during or just after exercise:

- Pain or pressure in the left or mid-chest area, left neck area, left shoulder, or left arm. The same goes for pain and tingling that radiates into the chin. Remember: Exercise is a stress test. If you feel these sensations during exercise, take that as a sign that your coronary arteries might not be functioning as they should.
- Loss of consciousness, dizziness, an irregular heartbeat, or extreme breathlessness, all of which may be side effects of medicines you are taking.

Dose: Ten to fifteen minutes two times a week. See my suggested strength training routine on pages 216 to 222.

Stretching. While stretching won't directly improve your heart health, it is important for your overall quality of life. It helps keep you active. More flexible, pliable muscles are less likely to get injured than tighter muscles. Plus, the more flexible you are, the better you feel. You'll be much less likely to suffer from chronic aches and pains such as back pain.

Dose: Ten minutes every day. Stretch after exercise or at the end of the day, when your muscles are warm and pliable. Try my suggested stretching routine on pages 222 to 223.

Before you try any of the routines suggested here, talk to your doctor about exercise to make sure you are ready. Especially make sure to talk to your doctor about medications and how they might interfere with exercise.

For example, you'll want to time your intake of beta-blockers so that your physical activity does not block the absorption of this medicine.

I highly recommend doing a cardiac rehabilitation program first, before starting your own fitness program. Cardiac rehabilitation will allow you to slowly improve your strength and stamina with the guidance of a therapist who is knowledgeable about heart disease.

How to Do Cardio

If you were a La-Z-Boy fan before your heart disease diagnosis, the idea of walking around the block a few times might seem about as enticing to you as the notion of eating a bowlful of your least favorite vegetable. That's okay. You are very normal. More important, you can overcome this inertia to move. All you need to do is move a little more, a little bit at a time. Take things one step at a time—literally, all the while using deep breathing to stay relaxed.

This is why most people hate to exercise: They do too much of it at once. As Americans we're conditioned to think of exercise and getting in shape as an all-or-nothing proposition. When we think about getting in shape, we think about Rocky Balboa running up the Art Museum steps in Philadelphia. We think of muscle aches and pain. We think about sweat and breathlessness.

It doesn't have to be that way! If you slowly ease yourself into fitness, it shouldn't hurt at all. And once you get past the initial inertia to move, you'll see that Newton's first law of motion is really true: A body in motion tends to stay in motion. You'll eventually come to enjoy moving. You'll not only like what it brings you—better health and a stronger, more capable body—you'll also like how it makes you feel. You'll appreciate the time to yourself and the time outdoors. Just like sex, you'll finish each session and say to yourself, "Wow, I feel really good right now. Why on Earth was I avoiding this?" Really, it's true. When it happens to you, you'll thank me.

My cardio plan includes two elements:

1. **Lifestyle movement.** This is how you move as you go about your day. To increase your lifestyle movement, you'll want to take the stairs instead of the elevator or escalator. Avoid any type of assisted movement, including moving walkways. Get out of the car whenever possible, too. Make it your goal to never use another drive-thru window again. If it's safe, always park in the first space you see, the one farthest from where you want to go. You'll probably find that this tactic will wind up saving you time, as you'll spend much less time sitting in your car as you circle the lot in search of a space. I do this all the time. It drives Jamie crazy, but it keeps us both moving.

    Keep in mind that you won't be able to tackle every type of lifestyle activity right away. Use this chart to gauge when you will be ready for certain types of activities after surgery. Whatever lifestyle activity you try, make sure not to force the issue. Don't push through pain and discomfort. Take your time and relax by taking deep breaths. Take breaks as needed.

Weeks 1 to 6

You can:

- Do light housekeeping such as dusting
- Set the table

- Wash dishes
- Fold clothes
- Pot plants
- Trim flowers
- Walk short distances

After 6 Weeks

You can:

- Vacuum lightly
- Sweep the floor gently
- Carry, fold, and do laundry in general
- Cut the grass without much force and in small amounts at a time
- Walk the dog on a leash

After 3 Months

You can:

- Scrub floors
- Garden
- Shovel
- Rake leaves
- Play sports (such as soccer, baseball, tennis)

2. **Daily cardio.** You can do any form of cardiovascular exercise you like, including cycling, swimming, running, and more. If you hate to exercise, however, I encourage you to start with walking because it's the

most accessible form of exercise around. All you need is your body and a good pair of shoes to make it happen. You can walk anywhere: malls, outside, and even hallways. It's an excuse-proof form of exercise.

Use this advice:

Start with what you can handle and gradually increase your distance. A good rule of thumb is to add about 10 percent to your longest session each week.

Warm up before each session and cool down after each session with lower-intensity movement. Slow walking will allow you to gradually speed up and decrease your heart rate.

Don't exercise right after eating. Exercising on a full stomach is uncomfortable for anyone. Our bodies are not as efficient at digesting food during exercise. During exercise the body shuttles some of your blood flow away from your digestive tract and toward your working muscles. As a result, digestion comes to a halt, and this sensation just doesn't feel all that comfortable if there is partially digested food sitting in your stomach or intestines. Therefore, overeating prior to a workout can make you feel sluggish and can cause stomach cramps.

Pay attention to the weather. Know that extreme temperatures and humidity will not just tire you more quickly, but also possibly trigger chest pain and interfere with circulation. Very hot or very cold weather can be especially fatiguing when you have heart disease. On extremely cold and hot days, exercise indoors, either at a gym on a treadmill, at home, or at a mall. I do this quite often so I don't have to worry about the extremes of weather. The treadmill has become a friend.

Drink plenty of water. This is especially important on hot days. Have a glass before you set out on a walk and another when you return. I carry water everywhere, even when I am not exercising. Remember, it is very important to prime the pump while you are being refreshed.

Go flat and easy. Until you've increased your fitness, avoid hilly walking routes. Hills will tax you, speeding up your heart rate. It's good to include some hills eventually, but avoid them in the beginning. As a general rule, focus on duration first—getting your daily walks up to at least thirty minutes. Then you can up the intensity, either by including some hills or by trying faster walking or running.

Do it with someone you love. A partner can offer support, motivate you, and help soothe your fears when, say, you go out a little farther than your comfort level. If you do not have family members or friends who you feel comfortable asking to accompany you, then look for a walking partner online. Look into the American Heart Association's MyStart! community, an online social network for people who are trying to increase their physical activity through walking. You'll find contact information for this organization in Chapter 13. This site also has a handy online tracker that maps out your distance traveled.

Reward yourself for reaching specific milestones. As you accomplish your fitness goals, reward yourself for a job well done. Once you can walk a mile, for instance, consider treating yourself to a healthy dinner out at your favorite restaurant, a weekend away, or a new pair of shoes. As I was getting back into shape, such rewards were very important to me. They made me feel wonderful and gave me an incentive to continue.

How to Strength Train

Strength train one to two times a week. If you have a set of exercises from cardiac rehabilitation, do those. If not, try this total-body-fitness plan. It works all the major muscle groups. You'll find options for a home-based routine as well as a gym routine. If you are using weights at the gym, start with the lightest weight that you can comfortably lift. Slowly increase the weight over time, until the last two repetitions of any given exercise feel very challenging.

Note: Only do this routine if your blood pressure is under control. If your blood pressure is above normal, consult your doctor, as certain weight-training movements can cause blood pressure to spike temporarily. For this reason, it's very important to remember to breathe as you lift, exhaling during the hardest part of the lift and inhaling during the easier part. Holding your breath and straining will boost your pressure. Ideally, these exercises should be started slowly, under the watchful eye of a trained professional, and should not start until your cardiologist says you are ready.

Exercise #1: Chest

It's important to strengthen your chest area, but you need to tackle this slowly and safely. This area of your body will be very weak if you underwent bypass surgery. In order to gain access to your heart, your surgeon sliced through your chest bone and weakened your chest muscles. It will take some work to get them back into shape. This is why I suggest you strengthen your chest in stages. Do one of the following exercises, based on your level of fitness and whether or not you have access to a gym.

Plank: Get in a push-up position with your hands on the floor under your shoulders and your arms and legs extended. Hold for up to 60 seconds. Once you can hold for 60 seconds, advance to the push-up.

Push-up: Start from a modified plank position with your knees on the floor. Slowly lower your chest to the floor. Once you are an inch or two from the floor, push back up. Once you can do 12 push-ups with your knees on the floor, try a standard push-up with your legs extended. Once you can do 12 standard push-ups, advance to the chest press.

Note: If you have wires in your chest, do not lower all the way to the floor in a strict military push-up. Just go down as far as you can comfortably, then press back up.

Chest press: This is similar to a push-up with weights. Lie on your back. Extend your arms at chest level. Lower the weights to your chest and then press them back up.

If you have access to a gym, you can do this in a chest press machine or under a Smith machine (a barbell attached to steel rails). Both will allow you to lift weights safely, without worrying about getting stuck under a bar or not being able to push the weight back up. If you don't have access to a gym, you can do a chest press at home with dumbbells, either by lying on the floor (least effective) or some sort of a bench (most effective). If you don't have a traditional weight bench, try placing a towel over a piano bench or a picnic table bench.

Whether you do the chest press at home or at the gym, perform 12 repetitions.

Note: If you have wires in your chest, don't lower the weight all the way to your chest, and have someone spot you for safety. Even more crucial, it is important to let a trained professional teach you these exercises.

Exercise #2: Upper Back

Strengthening your upper back will help improve your posture. Choose one exercise below, depending on whether you are exercising at home or at a gym.

At home: Do a reverse plank. Sit on the ground with your legs slightly bent. Place your palms on the floor just behind your buttocks. Keep your knees bent as you lift your buttocks, forming a table position with your body. Hold up to 30 seconds.

Once you can hold for a full 30 seconds, advance to the full reverse plank by extending your legs so your body forms a straight diagonal line from your feet to your head.

At the gym: Use the lat pull-down machine, bringing to bar to your collarbones. Do 12 repetitions.

Exercise #3: Shoulders

Strengthening your shoulders will both improve your posture and make objects easier to lift. Choose one of the following options, based on your level of fitness and whether you are exercising at home or at the gym.

Home option #1: If you do not have equipment, do the downward-facing dog yoga pose. Start on your hands and knees. Press into your palms as you raise your buttocks toward the ceiling. Rest your head between your arms, lift your tailbone (like a dog with a "happy tail"), and lower your heels if possible, bringing your body into an upside-down V. Hold up to 60 seconds. Release.

Home option #2: If you have dumbbells, do a shoulder press. Sit on a chair. Raise the dumbbells to shoulder height with your palms facing forward. Extend your arms as you raise the dumbbells. Then lower and repeat, completing 15 repetitions.

Gym option: Do a shoulder press. You can do this either by using the shoulder press machine or by using dumbbells. For dumbbells, sit on the edge of a bench. Raise the dumbbells to shoulder height with your palms facing forward. Extend your arms as you raise the dumbbells. Then lower and repeat, completing 15 repetitions.

Exercise #4: Triceps

Your triceps are the muscles in the back of your upper arms. Stronger triceps allow you to more easily support your body weight, for instance as you ease yourself into or out of a pool. Choose one of the following options, depending on whether you will be exercising at home or at a gym.

At home: Do chair dips. Sit on the edge of a sturdy chair, one that does not have wheels. Rest your palms on either side of your buttocks. Scoot your buttocks off the chair. Bend your elbows as you lower your buttocks. Once your upper arms are parallel to the floor, press back up to the starting position. Do 10 to 12 repetitions.

At the gym: Try the triceps press-down. Use the triceps press-down cable. Grasp the bar with your palms facing down. Keep your elbows in close to your torso as you press the bar down. Then slowly allow the bar to rise to the starting position. Do 10 to 12 repetitions.

Exercise #5: Biceps

To work your biceps at home, you'll eventually need a set of dumbbells. Initially, large cans of food or frozen water bottles might be heavy enough to do the trick. You can do the same dumbbell exercise at the gym, or you can use the biceps machine.

To do biceps curls with dumbbells, sit in a chair or on the edge of a bench. Grasp the dumbbells in each hand and extend your arms to the ground. Raise one hand at a time toward your upper arm, then lower and repeat on the other side. Alternate sides for 10 to 12 repetitions on each side.

Exercise #6: Legs

Lunges are a great leg exercise that works everything at once. You can do lunges both at home and at the gym. Stand normally with your feet hip-distance apart. Step forward about two to three feet with your right foot. Bend both knees and sink down, until both knees form right angles to the floor. Press back up and return to the starting position. Do 10 to 15 lunges with your right leg. Then switch to your left leg and repeat.

Exercise #7: Abs

You can do crunches both at home and at the gym, but start slowly and ease into them, especially if your chest still hurts. Lie with your knees bent and the soles of your feet on the ground. Place your hands behind your head, with your elbows open to the side. Use your abdomen to lift your shoulders and upper back. Exhale as you rise and inhale as you lower. Lower and repeat 15 times.

Exercise #8: Lower Back

You can do the reciprocal reach at home and at the gym. Kneel on all fours. Extend your right arm and left leg. Hold for a count of 5. Lower and then repeat with your left arm and right leg. Continue alternating sides until you've completed 10 repetitions on each side.

Again, remember that these exercises need to be taught so that you are careful even if you have been doing them for years. Start with a certified trainer before you do anything on your own.

How to Stretch

I recommend you stretch every day. Your muscles tend to tighten within twenty-four hours if you don't. Stretch just after exercise or at the end of the day, when your muscles are warm. If you have a set of stretches from your cardiac rehabilitation plan, do those. If not, use these:

Wall push: Stand facing a wall. Place both palms on the wall. Slightly bend one knee while extending the other leg behind you. Press into your hands and press both heels to the floor, leaning into the wall until you feel a stretch in your back calf. Hold about 15 to 20 seconds, until your muscle feels warm and loose. Then switch legs and repeat.

Back extensions: Only do this stretch once you've fully recovered from surgery. Lie on your belly. Place your palms on the floor, just in front of your shoulders. Press into your palms as you lift your torso, arching your back as far as you can comfortably. Hold for a count of 5, lower, and repeat for a total of 10 repetitions.

Chest stretch: Clasp your hands behind your back. Lift your arms as high as you can comfortably. Hold 15 to 20 seconds. Lower and repeat one time.

Hip stretch: Sit with your legs crossed. Lean forward as far as you can comfortably. Hold 15 to 20 seconds. Rise and repeat with your legs crossed in the opposite direction (with the opposite leg on top or in front).

Hamstring stretch: Lie on your back. Lift one leg, placing the middle of a towel around that foot and holding one end of the towel in each hand. Extend that leg toward the ceiling. Use the towel to gently pull your leg toward you until you feel a stretch. Hold 15 to 20 seconds. Release and repeat with the other leg.

How to Challenge Yourself

Once you are in shape, it's time to start thinking about that challenge—the physical feat that will prove to you and others that you are back and ready to tackle any problem that comes your way.

Simply put, your challenge is the one thing you most fear doing. Before my illness, the marathon was a milestone. It was proof that the human body was capable of extraordinary feats. It was an achievement. Each finish line made me feel invincible.

And then, in a matter of moments, heart disease made me feel so vulnerable that I wasn't even sure whether or not I could go to sleep without dying, walk down the street without dying, make love to my wife without dying, or withstand the everyday stress of my career without dying.

Yes, my doctor did test after test to prove to me that my newly bypassed arteries were working, that my heart was getting plenty of blood, and that I was cured. I'd had the stress tests and echocardiograms, but I needed more.

I needed the marathon. I needed to prove to myself that I could conquer the distance again. I needed to prove to myself that I was strong and healthy, that I was *not* going to die by doing something as mundane as walking up a flight of stairs. If I could run another marathon, there was nothing my heart could not withstand.

I, again, would have that wonderful feeling of being on top of the world, of being invincible.

At the same time, I was scared.

This, I knew, was normal. Even the most successful athletes and CEOs question whether they will reach their goals. The most successful fail, many times. They, too, have doubts and fears, but they keep trying. They continually challenge themselves until they succeed, one challenge at a time.

I hoped to follow in their footsteps.

Your challenge might not be a marathon, as it was for me, but it's also not knitting, crossword puzzles, the jumble, or poker. I'm talking about something physical, not about something mental. I'm talking about getting your heart rate up. I'm talking about walkathons, marathons, triathlons, long-distance cycling, adventure races, survivalist outings, and long-distance backpacking excursions. I'm talking about doing the thing that you most love but also most fear. It has to be something that gets you moving and is considered aerobic exercise, with walking distances being the most practical and least stressful.

Pick the biggest, baddest, scariest feat that exists in your world. Once you tackle it, nothing will ever feel as scary again. Remember Tony Soprano. You are going after your personal bodyguard!

Pick a challenge that is:

Realistic but scary. Some change is good, but too much change can be paralyzing. You want something that will make you proud, but not something so hard that you feel immobilized just thinking about it. Be honest with yourself in coming up with realistic yet challenging goals. If you did not exercise before your diagnosis, a good first goal might be a three-mile walk. If you were very fit before your diagnosis, it might be something much more challenging. Pick a goal that will prove to the most doubtful part of yourself that you are alive and will continue to be for a long time to come. You need a goal that gives you hope. Only you can find the right balance.

Measurable. You need to know when you've accomplished your goal. If you want to become more active, define what you mean by that in a specific and measurable way. Do you want to exercise for thirty minutes three times a week? That's measurable. Do you want to run a 5K? That's measurable—you cross the finish line and you've reached your goal.

Meaningful. You'll have an easier time staying motivated if your challenge speaks to a deep part of yourself. Choose a physical challenge that defines you. Ed Hommer decided to climb Mount McKinley because it was the same mountain his plane flew into, an accident that caused him to lose his feet. After surviving intense chemotherapy to treat testicular cancer, Lance Armstrong chose the Tour de France because he was a professional cyclist and the tour represents the pinnacle cycling achievement. Ardell Lien, a seventy-one-year-old heart and kidney transplant patient, sailed

✦ THE UNBEATABLES ✦

Don Monroe was a runner and a high school track and cross-country coach.
He was fit and healthy. He wasn't the type of person you would expect to
get heart disease. But he did. The first symptoms hit during his runs, when
he noticed that he did not have the endurance or energy he'd once had.
Then, during one run, he felt pain between his shoulder blades. He told his
wife about it. She knew about his family history—particularly about his two
uncles who had died of heart attacks before age forty. She suggested he see
a doctor. He learned that his coronary arteries were blocked, and that he
would need a bypass. Here's how he reclaimed his life.

———

I'd just turned fifty when I had my bypass. I had three marathons behind
me. My biggest fear after my diagnosis was not about the surgery itself.
It was about running. I loved running and I worried that I might not be
able to do it again.

My biggest problem after my surgery? Impatience. I wanted to get
back to running and back to coaching. My rehabilitation therapist had
to put the reins on me and slow me down. It took about eight to twelve
months before I was back on my feet again and could run three to five
miles a day and return to coaching.

Although I've come back, I've had to learn to accept the fact that I
am not the runner or the coach I once was. With my coaching, for
instance, I realized that I could no longer keep up with the kids like I
used to do. I had the endurance but not the speed. Instead of running
the workouts with them, I had to coach them from the sidelines.

Before my diagnosis, I thought my running could take care of any
indiscretions I took with my diet. That, of course, was not true, so after

my diagnosis I made some changes. I stopped drinking soft drinks. I put an end to my morning routine of stopping at a local doughnut shop on my way to work. I cut back on red meat.

In place of the soft drinks, I started drinking water, milk, and tea. In place of the junk food, I began eating more fruits and vegetables. I swapped my nightly cheese and crackers for carrots.

I also learned to be thankful for what the disease taught me, particularly about the importance of my family in my life. My wife and daughter were very supportive during my recovery. My daughter even came and stayed with us for a while. My brothers helped out, too. I'm thankful that I had the opportunity to grow closer to them all.

Don's Unbeatable Advice: Set a goal for yourself. My goal was returning to coaching. Yours might be something else. It should be something you can look forward to as you recover. It's important to have something to strive for, something that you can go after and enjoy.

solo around the world—accomplishing a lifelong dream and becoming the first heart and kidney recipient to accomplish the feat.

In my case, it had to be the marathon. There was no question about it. I'd run six marathons and four half-marathons before my surgery, and I needed to run one after it to prove to myself that I was healthy and fit again.

If nothing immediately comes to mind, consider doing a heart-disease-related challenge. For instance, you might look into signing up for a Start! Heart Walk. Sponsored by the American Heart Association, these walks raise money to help fight heart disease and are held at various locations around the country. Check the resources section in Chapter 13 for information on heart-disease-themed events.

Public. Research has shown that making a goal public raises your chances of success. When you keep a goal a secret, it's just too easy to call it quits or change it on a whim. When the going gets tough, you might ask yourself, "Did I really want to run a marathon? No, I wanted to run a 10K." Tell at least one other person about your goal. The person you tell can offer you emotional support as well as keep you accountable to your goal. In addition to telling one other person, write it down, for the same reason. It will keep you accountable.

If your goal is extremely personal, the person you tell may be someone anonymous whom you meet in an Internet chat room or it might be a therapist or pastor. Be creative. You can also make your goal public by lining up some support. If you have the means, hire a coach or trainer to help get you physically ready. If money is an issue, look for a training group or club for guidance. I kept no secrets about my comeback plan. I told anyone who would listen, but I only did so once I was fully committed and had a race on the calendar, which was about three months before the actual event.

Pick your goal and commit yourself to it. Sign up for a specific date. Tell others, and then move on to Step 2.

Step 2: Create a Training Plan

By June 2004, the New York City marathon was just a few months away. A nurse who'd been in the operating room during my surgery—someone who had both seen my heart and who knew I ran—asked me one day, "Are you going to run New York?"

I said, "I'm not sure. I'm not sure I'm ready. I don't have anyone to train me."

She introduced me to her husband, Neil Cook, who had trained the rap star P. Diddy to finish the New York City marathon the year before. Now it was getting serious. Now I had a coach. He helped me go from wanting to run a marathon to doing it. He created the training plan, the step-by-step program that got me to the marathon's start.

Either with the help of a coach or on your own, create a plan, a step-by-step guide that will get you to your goal. Without a plan, you will wander aimlessly and wind up stuck where you are. Your training plan should include more than just your workouts. You'll need to plan how you will make the time and energy to get it all done. Do you need to ask for more support at home? When will you train and where? If your only free time is in the evenings, perhaps you should invest in a gym membership so you don't have to train in the dark.

Also try to think about possible problems that might arise, and solve them before you start training. For instance, if you are training for a cycling event, what will you do on days when the weather prevents you from riding outdoors? A possible solution would be setting up your bike indoors on a stationary trainer, watching movies as you ride, or joining a spinning class.

You can also try cross-training, perhaps by using the stair stepper, elliptical trainer, or rowing machine at your gym. You will still get an aerobic workout, and the cross-training can help prevent repetitive-strain injuries.

In Chapter 13, on pages 283 to 292, you will find specific training plans for some common challenges. No matter the type of challenge you pick, use this training advice:

Start with the shortest race distance possible. For example, if you've never gone farther than a mile, then the 5K is your race. If you did 5Ks and 10Ks before your event, then go for the 10K, and so on. Don't tackle the longest race imaginable first.

Make it your goal to finish. Don't try to finish your first challenge within a set amount of time. I, for one, had no time in mind. I just wanted to cross the finish line. That was it. This is especially important if you've never before completed a given distance. You will face a variety of emotional and physical hurdles during your training—hurdles that you've never before faced. Your body may feel foreign to you—it might not respond to the type of training and pace that you were once used to. You might feel extremely cold or extremely hot and have to find creative ways to manage your body temperature.

This first challenge will establish a new personal best for you. Once you establish this new best time, you can make it your goal in your next race to race for time and break this initial record. Again, after your first race, you'll know what you can handle, and you can up the ante and train even harder to finish your second race even more quickly. For now, back off, enjoy the journey, and reach the finish line.

Train just enough. You'll notice that the training plans in Chapter 13 do not include a heck of a lot of training. Many of them have just three sessions a week. I've designed these plans for beginners and busy professionals. This minimal training approach is just enough to build your fitness, but not so much that you will feel overwhelmed, get injured, or burn out. Remember: Even if it's a full two years after open-heart surgery or a heart attack, your heart is a muscle that needs time to grow stronger. It needs a combination of exercise and rest. It needs time to wake up and get back in shape. Resist the urge to get in shape in just one day (sometimes called New Year's Resolutioner's Syndrome). Working out for an hour or more every day without a break will not necessarily get you in shape any faster than my minimal training approach. My approach provides the necessary rest, and won't burn you out.

Get good shoes. Shoes are your most important pieces of equipment for walking, running, hiking, and many other adventures you take on your feet. A good pair will cost you about $100 (more if you are looking for hiking boots). If you've never before purchased running or walking shoes, I highly recommend visiting a quality athletic shoe store, the type where experts fit you with shoes and offer to watch your form as you walk and run in them. Once you have a pair that works for you, it's okay to purchase subsequent pairs online or at discount stores. If you want to invest more, look into performance apparel, especially if your race will be in a very hot or very cold environment. These synthetic outfits are wonders. They wick sweat away from your skin, dry quickly, and weigh almost nothing. They keep you warm in the winter and dry and cool in the summer.

Train with others. It's simple: Training buddies help you stay motivated. If you have to meet someone for a workout session, you'll be that much less likely to say, "Oh, I'm too busy to do this today." More important, your buddies can encourage you, help you solve problems, and make the time go by more quickly. Look into local running and walking clubs, do it with a friend, sign up for a charity event that offers training support (many Team In Training events do this), or hire a coach.

Monitor your heart rate. During training, I recommend that you keep your heart rate in the neighborhood of 30 beats above your resting heart rate (your pulse first thing in the morning), especially in the beginning. Once you are sure of your fitness, you can push it a bit harder. If in doubt, ask your cardiologist about how much to exert yourself.

If you walk, run, hike, or cycle, you can monitor your effort by using a heart-rate monitor. You wear a strap around your chest, which communicates information to your watch, allowing you to easily check your heart rate at any given time. I always wear one.

If you can't afford a heart-rate monitor, monitor your pulse every mile (or every fifteen minutes) or so. To take your pulse, place your index and middle fingers on the lower part of your thumb, then slide your fingers down to your wrist. If you do not feel the pulse, try moving your fingers over a little bit in the same area. Once you can feel the pulse, count it for fifteen seconds and multiply by four. This will tell you how many times your heart is beating in one minute. Always remember that these plans must be done in conjunction with both approval from and careful monitoring by your cardiologist.

Step 3: Follow Your Plan

Once a week Neil met me at Central Park. He rode his bike beside me as I ran, all the while asking me, "How are you feeling? What is in your head? What are you thinking about?"

Each week the runs got longer. Each week Neil helped me confront my fears. I had so many of them. We tackled my fear of running in Central Park, the same place where I'd experienced the angina that led to my diagnosis. We tackled my fear of running uphill, of having my heart rate speed up. He even trained me through my fear of running in crowds.

A few weeks before the marathon, I ran three hours through Central Park as he rode by my side. I finished that run feeling normal, like myself again. I finished knowing that I had returned, that I was back. I finished knowing that I could continue to define myself by running marathons.

As you train, expect the unexpected. You may have to confront many unusual fears and situations in order to complete your training. For instance, I experienced an angina episode while running outside. After my bypass, the treadmill became a security blanket for me. Unfortunately, you can't run marathons on treadmills! I had to get over my fear of running outdoors.

Use this advice:

Confront your fear when you are most able. Tackle hills and other scary feats for the first time on your easy days. Don't do your first hill on the day you are also doing your longest effort!

Keep your loved ones informed. They may not automatically be supportive. Remember, your loved ones are scared, too. My trainer periodically called my wife from his cell phone on our training runs just to say, "Marc's okay. He's doing fine." Take your loved ones with you to your doctor's appointments, so they can hear your doctor give you clearance to challenge yourself physically.

Keep a training log or a diary. Write down all the training you complete, along with how you felt (good, bad, bored, on top of the world, achy, scared etc.). Understand that some training sessions will be easier to accomplish than others. If needed, review your training diary with a coach or physician to help solve potential training problems. Your training diary is also a great confirmation of who you are becoming. Read it over every so often to see just how dramatically you are reinventing yourself.

Continually motivate yourself. As you train—and especially as the training gets more and more challenging—it's important to keep yourself motivated. Try the following:

- Read a book or watch a video (if possible) about the challenge, or about someone else attempting a similar challenge. For instance, I found Lance Armstrong's *It's Not About the Bike* incredibly motivating as I was training for my marathon.
- Watch a race. Go to a walkathon, 10K, endurance bike ride, or some other race that is similar to the challenge you wish to attempt. Cheer for the participants, especially those who are trudging through that final, hard stretch of the race before the finish line (usually miles 20 to 26 in a marathon). Soak up the crowd support, too. During my recovery, I watched two New York City marathons from the sidelines. It gave me both the courage and motivation to, that third year, be one of the runners.

Step 4: Measure and Reassess

This is the step so many people skip, yet it's essential to your success. Periodically you need to find out whether your training is getting you closer to your goal. Can you progressively work out longer or faster from week to week?

Setbacks are inevitable when pursuing a long-term goal, so remember to be flexible and not to get discouraged if you don't always meet your daily goals. Try to see setbacks as problems that, with enough creativity, you can solve.

At some point during your training, you'll want to quit. You'll do a workout that feels incredibly hard and you'll say to yourself, "There's no way I can do this." Let's say you are training for a marathon. You'll do that first long run—the 17- to 20-miler—and hit the wall mentally and physically. It will take everything you have to get through it. You'll think to yourself, "This workout is the hardest thing I've ever done. How will I ever do more?"

I have five words for you: You can and you will.

When you feel overwhelmed, remind yourself how far you've come. Before you ever took a step, you probably never thought you could do what you did today. Remind yourself that this really hard workout not only trained your physical body, it also trained your mind. Remind yourself that you've gotten clearance from your physician. If needed, call or visit your doctor again to improve your confidence in your abilities. And remind yourself why you are doing this. I liked to remind myself that this was the way I was celebrating the next chapter of my life.

Also, try to focus on the moment, on putting one foot in front of the other.

If things get and stay hard without a break, assess whether training for your goal is working. Exercise is the best stress test there is. Notice any sensations in your chest and mention them to your doctor. The same goes for a twinge in your knee or any other area of your body. If you ignore aches and pains, just one thing will happen: You will have aches and pains even more! Most important, if you feel very tired consistently, that's a sign that you are overtraining. It is critical that you get enough rest. Back off and rest more. It doesn't matter if it takes you twice as long to complete your training plan as long as you eventually get to the finish line.

Here's another sign that your training isn't working: You are losing touch with other important aspects of your life. If you are getting one cold after another along with intense knee pain, and your spouse and kids are complaining that they never see you, then you need to reassess your training and/or your goal. You must keep your entire life full, not just one aspect of it. Everyone in your life needs to be on board. This should be an empowering experience for all of you.

Step 5: Role Play

Your big goal may involve many scary and anxiety-producing variables. For example, when I wanted to run the marathon, I not only had to conquer the distance, I also had to conquer my fear of running in a crowd. I had to find the courage to run the same path and incline where I'd felt the chest pain that led to my bypass. Rather than deal with all those fears on the same day, I retraced my steps before the marathon. I did a lot of my running outdoors, in Central Park, in the very place where I was most afraid. Perhaps most important, I did a test run before the marathon. I ran a 5K. It helped me get used to the race atmosphere before my big day. You may not be able to play out some aspect of every type of goal, but with some creativity you can probably simulate the experience for many of them.

Step 6: Reach Your Goal

Do what you set out to do. Don't beat yourself up if it takes more than one attempt.

Step 7: Set a New Goal

What will you do next? What does the third part of your life have in store for you?

For me, the next goal was simple. I ran another marathon. Then things got more complicated. I *could* have continued to run marathons. Yet I felt pulled to challenge myself in new ways. So I trained for and finished a triathlon; I had not been swimming since summer camp!

If at all possible, set your next goal before you reach your current goal. If you are running a marathon, sign up for the next race before finishing the current one. That way you won't backslide. You'll have something to propel yourself forward. These goals are critical to show that you are alive and invested. They help you say to your inner doubter, "I am still around, and I will keep showing up!"

❋   BACK TO LIFE R$_x$ ❋

- As soon as you are ready, pick one challenge that is meaningful, one that will prove to your biggest inner critic that you can do anything.
- Train for it in baby steps.
- Cross the finish line.
- Celebrate.
- Repeat.

❖ PART THREE ❖

The Support

11

The Finish Line

MARATHON DAY WAS BEAUTIFUL. THE SKY WAS CLEAR. THE TEMPERA-
ture was warm. Could I do it? Could I really conquer this distance again? I
reminded myself of the stories of many other marathoners. Heart transplant patients ran marathons. Cancer survivors ran marathons. People
with multiple sclerosis ran marathons. People with artificial limbs ran
marathons. If they could do it, so could I.

I could do this. I could finish this.

My first test came, as I expected, on the Verrazano-Narrows Bridge
between Staten Island and Brooklyn. It's two miles long, and the first mile
is uphill. I knew the bridges would test me. I knew my heart rate would go
up on the hill. I knew the race would be very crowded at that point. I knew
I would have to confront many fears to get myself over that bridge.

I was running with a heart-rate monitor, as I had done during all my training runs. It gave me confidence about what my heart could and couldn't do. It had become a security blanket of sorts. As I climbed the initial hill on that bridge, the readout on the monitor told me that my heart rate had gone up to 150 beats per minute. I thought, "I'm not sure I'm going to be able to do this. What was I thinking?"

Neil was running next to me. He slowed me down to a walk. He started talking: "You've trained for such a long time. This is so important to you. Relax. Your heart is fine. This is all anxiety. Take some deep breaths. Let's see if you can get yourself relaxed and over this bridge."

He was right. My heart rate hadn't spiked because I could not handle the hill. It had spiked because I didn't believe I could handle the hill. Once I relaxed and took some deep breaths, it lowered to 110 beats per minute. We picked up the pace and began to run again.

Later, on flat ground through city streets, my heart rate again started to climb. "It's early in the race," I thought. "I shouldn't be laboring this much so early in the race. What's wrong? What am I doing wrong? I am drinking plenty of fluids. I'm running at a slow pace. What am I doing wrong?"

Neil read my thoughts and asked, "What are you doing wrong?"

I said, "I don't know."

He said, "Look ahead of you. Look at the runners ahead of you. What are they doing that you are not doing? Let me ask you something. Do you feel hot?"

I looked ahead. The other runners were all on one side of the street. I was on the other. They were running in the shade. I was in the sun. I started running in the shade to cool down. My heart rate slowed.

I faced many more fears and challenges along the way. There were more bridges to cross with long hills and traffic. There were times when I told myself, "If I can just get to mile 14, that will be enough for today. If I can just get to mile 17, that will be enough for today. If I can just get to . . ."

The race route would go by my apartment. Many, many times, I thought, "If I can just get to Seventy-second Street and First Avenue in Manhattan, I can walk home from there."

But by the time I got to Seventy-second Street, I was feeling great. I saw Jamie. I said, "I'm going to finish this."

Neil's wife, Julie, the nurse who had assisted my heart surgeon, took over the job of coaching and pacing me once we got to Central Park. She'd already finished the race and had jogged back to find me and bring me to the finish line. We went up and down the hills of the park, and I battled the usual fatigue that most marathoners battle during those last grueling miles. I still had that thought, "I am not sure I can finish this," but all the while Julie was there, telling me, "You are almost there. This is ridiculous. You can't quit now!"

When I got to Central Park South, I had just one mile to go. I heard the crowds cheering me and the other runners on. It was then that I knew I would make it. I knew I would be able to finish.

I crossed the finish line. The surgery really had worked. My arteries really were open, with plenty of blood flowing through them and into my heart. I really was healthy. I really could handle anything—even a marathon— without dropping dead. My heart rate had gone up to 150 beats per minute during the race, and nothing had happened!

In that moment, I knew I'd reclaimed my life. One phrase came to mind. It was, "I'm back. I can do anything."

I initially was against Marc running. I worried about his health. Once his training progressed and his appearance, posture, mood, attitude, and even his sense of humor improved, it was unmistakable. This quest was helping him reclaim his life.

Encourage your loved one to pace him or herself, but don't assume that he or she can't accomplish this physical goal. Be your partner's greatest cheerleader.

I know I tried my best. I couldn't be with Marc all 26.2 miles, so I made a shirt with "Go, Marc" on it. As Marc ran, people saw the shirt, called his name, and encouraged him. They cheered him on for me.

And Life Went On

About a year after my marathon, my mother became very ill and was admitted to Metropolitan Hospital, where I now work. Not long after, she died. Then my brother became ill and passed away, too.

These were tough times for me. Still, had I not finished the marathon that day, they would have been even tougher. Had I not finished the marathon that day, I would not have had the faith to keep on living, no matter the adversity. I would not have felt—Jamie's dad, Marty Colby, always tells me I am—invincible. I would not have assumed that I could handle any situation life brought my way. I would have lived the rest of my life afraid.

Had I not finished the marathon that day, I would have still doubted myself. I would have still felt weak. I would have still had that fear of the unknown, of not knowing whether I was strong enough to endure.

The marathon taught me that life could, indeed, continue.

Gone was the deadly fear of death. Gone was the worry that the book of my life would forever go unfinished, that my "the end" would come too soon, before I had a chance to pen all the chapters that came in the middle. Gone was the bargaining for one more day. Gone were the haunting thoughts of personal and professional frailties. Gone were the worries that my life and career would be a tragic footnote in a greater story.

The fear was gone. All that remained was hope. My life began a new chapter, one that I could not wait to experience.

Your Book of Life

Once you cross that initial finish line, you will know that there is nothing that you cannot do. To succeed at anything in life—at work, at home, in hobbies, in friendships—you just need to set a goal and create a training plan to get you from point A to point B. By training for that goal—by putting one foot in front of the other over and over again—you grow stronger, healthier, and happier. You gain confidence. You overcome your fears and doubts. You become invincible.

The finish line is not an ending. It's a beginning, the beginning of the rest of your life.

I try to set and reach a new goal each year. Each time I set a new goal, I must further confront the fear within me. Each finish line makes me feel more alive, confident, and complete. It's a long road just to cross the starting line, and an even longer one to each finish. Anything can kick me and try to knock me down. No matter what, as long as my heart is still beating, I will get up and I will put one foot in front of the other, and I will run.

Today, whenever I get dressed, I see the scar on my chest. It reminds

me of the fragility of life. It reminds me that life could end in an instant, in a footstep, in a stride during any training run. I use this reminder to live every moment to the fullest, as if it were my last.

❀   **BACK TO LIFE R$_x$**   ❀

- Consult backtolifethebook.com for support, help, and motivation as often as needed. I'll be updating the site regularly with new tips, recipes, my own personal milestones, and more Unbeatable stories.
- Become an Unbeatable. Write your comeback story and send it to me at info@backtolifethebook.com to be included with other Unbeatable stories on our site. Let your success inspire others.
- Share your expertise. Send your favorite heart-healthy recipes and advice to me at info@backtolifethebook.com. We'll include it on our site, so other survivors can learn from your experience.

12

The Back-to-Life Recipe Collection

MANY YEARS BEFORE MY HEART DISEASE DIAGNOSIS, I VISITED THE Canyon Ranch health spa in Tucson, Arizona. The trip was partly a vacation, but I also used it to learn more about proper nutrition. It was there that I learned how to follow a low-fat, medium-carbohydrate, lean-protein diet. Over the years, I've taken what I learned there a step further, adapting the nutrition advice for someone with heart disease.

I visited and taught at the Canyon Ranch every year for about eight years afterward. The visits helped Jamie and me recommit to the diet and exercise plan I needed to follow.

Throughout the following pages, you'll find many of the delicious recipes Jamie and I have developed over the years and still enjoy.

Jamie and I have found ways to enjoy heart-healthy eating, and you

They say everything in life happens for a reason. When I moved to New York, leaving my law practice and eventually ending up working on TV, one of my first on-air jobs was at the TV Food Network. I hosted five hundred cooking shows and developed healthy recipes for each one. I could never have known how valuable that job would prove to be.

If you are caring for someone who's had heart surgery, consider taking a cooking class. Learn how to cook in a healthier way. It may even be a class you can take together. As Marc says, "We are what we eat."

can, too. This recipe collection will show you how. The recipes in the following pages will teach you how to:

- Swap whole milk, cream, and butter for low-fat and nonfat ingredients— without sacrificing taste and texture.
- Keep chicken interesting!
- Cook vegetables that the entire family will want to eat.
- Sneak heart-healthy whole grains such as quinoa and brown rice into traditional favorites.
- Use delicious spices to flavor recipes, so you can cut down on the amount of sodium.

You'll find lots of comfort foods in here, too. We've tried to keep these recipes as simple, quick, and easy as possible, and we've tried to include fresh foods that require little prep time. The last thing you need to be doing as you are recovering from surgery is standing at a cutting board chopping, dicing, and slicing!

We also teach you how to bake some dishes rather than sauté them, which prevents you from having to stand at the stove for long periods of time. All told we've tried to keep everything as easy as possible, as delicious as possible, and as healthy as possible. Enjoy!

Phase I Recipes

During Phase 1, when you are feeling nauseous and have not one ounce of appetite, the last thing you want to eat for dinner is some sort of heart-healthy salad with wild salmon on top. So don't even try. Just get sustenance into your body in whatever form works, even if it's not the healthiest option around. You just need calories and protein. If you sneak a fruit or a vegetable in there—great. If not, don't sweat it. During Phase 1, Marc's diet included low-fat cottage cheese, applesauce, fat-free pudding, and other soft, easy-to-eat foods. Yours probably will as well.

The following recipes have all been designed with one purpose: to get food into your system during those initial days and weeks postsurgery. We've made sure they are easy to make, easy to eat (most are liquid), and easy to digest.

Smoothies

Smoothies are great for getting good nutrition into you without much fuss. Just make one in the morning and sip it over a period of hours.

Coffee Float

If you are suffering from those caffeine-withdrawal jitters, this is a recipe that you will soon come to love. Jamie used to make it for me as a special treat. I would look at her longingly each morning as she drank her coffee, until one day she took the last bit of her coffee and tossed it in a blender, inventing this wonderful drink.

MAKES 1 SERVING

½ cup vanilla or coffee nonfat ice cream or frozen yogurt

½ cup skim milk

2 tablespoons cold coffee

4 ice cubes

In a blender, combine the ice cream, milk, coffee, and ice cubes. Process until smooth, about 1 minute.

Strawberry Banana Smoothie

This traditional smoothie is loaded with all of the heart-healthy goodness fruit has to offer. The protein powder adds extra nutrients, especially on those days when you are not yet eating a well-balanced diet.

MAKES 2 SERVINGS (1 CUP EACH)

1 scoop vanilla-flavored protein powder

½ cup frozen strawberries

½ banana

½ cup skim milk

4 ice cubes

⊚ In a blender, combine all the ingredients. Process until smooth, 1 to 2 minutes. For extra calories you can always add orange or apple juice to a smoothie. Have fun. Don't be afraid to add stuff to your smoothie. It's all about calories at this point.

Soups

A bowl of soup can truly bring you back to your mother's kitchen, providing that nostalgic sense of warmth, comfort, and love. My grandmother and mother both made wonderful chicken soup, and they always made it with love. Whenever I ate it, I felt warm inside. It was an ambrosia of chicken, carrots, and celery.

If your appetite is small, as mine was those first few weeks, have soup as a meal unto itself. If you are slightly more hungry, serve it with a side of warm whole-grain bread. Once you have a heartier appetite, serve it as an appetizer before a main course.

The soup recipes in this section are low in fat and salt, two elements that you'll find in abundance in most commercial versions. They are based on a homemade Basic Chicken Stock (page 252). Although store-bought stock is easier, using homemade stock is the best way to control sodium without sacrificing flavor. This particular recipe calls for adding a little vinegar to the stock as it cooks, which helps extract extra calcium from the chicken bones.

If you wish to purchase a commercial soup or stock, opt for low-salt versions of vegetable, tomato, barley, or bean soup. Stay away from store-bought cream-based varieties, as most of these are made with butter and cream.

Basic Chicken Stock

Make this stock ahead of time, keeping some on hand at all times to make soup prep quick and easy. To store, allow it to cool, skim off any fat, cover, and store in the refrigerator for up to 10 days, or divide into 2-cup servings and freeze. For convenience, try freezing it in silicone muffin pans or ice cube trays, popping the frozen cubes into a zip-top freezer bag. As a general rule, each cube of stock melts down to about 2 tablespoons of stock (depending on the size of your ice cube trays), or about 1½ cups of stock per dozen cubes.

MAKES 12 CUPS STOCK, PLUS 4 CUPS COOKED CHICKEN

2 medium carrots, sliced

2 stalks celery, chopped

1 medium onion, quartered

2 teaspoons salt

Ground pepper, to taste

3 quarts cold water

4 pounds bone-in chicken breasts with skin

¼ cup white vinegar (optional)

Spray a large stockpot with cooking spray and place over medium heat. Add carrots, celery, onions, salt, and pepper and cook until translucent.

❀ Add water and chicken. Cover and continue to cook over medium heat. Add the vinegar, if using. Lower heat to simmer for approximately 1½ hours, skimming foam from the surface if it collects.

❀ Remove the chicken from the stock and, when cool enough to handle, discard the bones and skin. Save the chicken pieces for another use.

❀ Refrigerate overnight. Before using, discard any remaining fat that has hardened on the surface.

Chicken Noodle Soup

This will take you back to childhood, to a time when you felt warmth, comfort, and less fear.

MAKES 4 SERVINGS (1½ CUPS EACH)

1 tablespoon olive oil

1 teaspoon minced garlic

2 tablespoons finely chopped onion

½ teaspoon black pepper

1 carrot, chopped (about ½ cup)

4 cups reduced-sodium chicken broth or Basic Chicken Stock (page 252)

⅓ cup whole-grain pasta (see Note)

1 cup chopped cooked chicken

❀ Warm the oil in a 3½-quart pot over medium heat. Add the garlic, onion, and pepper, and cook for 30 seconds, until fragrant. Add the carrot and cook another 2 to 3 minutes, until the carrot begins to soften. Add the broth, pasta, and chicken. Bring to a boil and cook for 10 minutes, or until the pasta is al dente, or still slightly firm to the bite.

Note: Start with a small pasta, like a pastina, choosing larger shapes as your appetite increases.

Chinese Egg Drop Soup

This soup is rich in protein and flavor, and easy to prepare and digest. The ginger will warm your body and soul.

MAKES 2 SERVINGS (1 CUP EACH)

2 cups reduced-sodium chicken broth or Basic Chicken Stock (page 252)

½ teaspoon grated ginger (optional)

1 egg, lightly beaten

1 scallion, thinly sliced (about 1 tablespoon)

2 to 3 drops toasted sesame oil

Bring the broth or stock and optional ginger to a simmer in a small pot over high heat. Turn off the heat and give the stock a vigorous swirl. While the stock is moving, hold a fork above the pot and quickly pour the egg through the fork. Add the scallion and sesame oil, and stir to combine.

Phase 2 Recipes

Once you get past your initial recovery, it's time for some solid, old-fashioned comfort foods. The following recipes have adapted traditionally high-fat family favorites—meat loaf (page 263), macaroni and cheese (page 260), and tuna melt (page 262)—to make them good for your heart. They comfort you, bringing you back to that time, years ago, when you didn't have to worry about clogging your arteries.

If you don't see your personal comfort food favorites in this section, don't fret. You can adapt nearly any traditionally unhealthy favorite into a healthy one. Just use these simple substitutions:

- Nonfat or low-fat milk for whole milk. If thickness is important, use a combination of regular skim milk with evaporated skim milk.
- Low-fat cheese for regular cheese. Look for part-skim and low-fat versions of any regular cheese, or swap naturally lower-fat types of cheese—such as Parmesan and goat cheese—for higher-fat varieties. Or use less cheese in a recipe by switching to types with more flavor, such as extra-sharp cheddar, Gorgonzola, Parmesan, or Asiago.
- Substitute extra-lean beef, soy crumbles, or skinless or ground chicken or turkey breast for high-fat types of meat in any recipe.
- Jamie keeps olive oil in a spray bottle, the kind used for plants, and she can add flavor to any food without adding too much fat.

Breakfast Dishes

Breakfast doesn't have to be a production. A bowl of your favorite high-fiber, whole-grain cereal with skim milk or a piece of fruit with a slice of whole-grain toast is all you really need. My breakfast since my surgery and still today? Cheerios with fresh fruit and skim milk and two slices of whole-grain toast with Benecol spread or fat-free cream cheese. If you want a little something special in the morning—perhaps you're missing that morning stop at your local diner or doughnut shop—these recipes are for you.

Banana-Nut Muffins

The oats, banana, walnuts, and cranberries all add texture, flavor, and fiber to this delicious muffin favorite. The yogurt and nuts also increase the amount of protein.

MAKES 12 MUFFINS

1¼ cups rolled oats

1 cup all-purpose flour

2 teaspoons baking powder

½ cup dark brown sugar

1 large egg

¼ cup canola oil

1 very ripe banana, mashed (about ⅓ cup)

¼ cup vanilla yogurt

¾ cup chopped walnuts

¾ cup dried unsweetened cranberries or raisins

◉ Preheat the oven to 375°F. Coat a 12-cup muffin pan with cooking spray and set aside.

◉ Place the oats, flour, and baking powder in a medium bowl and stir until thoroughly combined. Set aside.

◉ In a large bowl, mix the brown sugar, egg, oil, and banana until smooth. Add the oat mixture and stir until thoroughly combined. Stir in the yogurt, followed by the walnuts and cranberries or raisins, mixing well after each addition.

◉ Fill the muffin cups two-thirds full and bake for 13 to 15 minutes, until the tops spring back lightly when touched. Loosen the sides with a knife, if necessary, and invert onto a wire rack to cool.

Roasted Sweet Potato Hash

Roasting intensifies the sweetness of sweet potatoes, so we've balanced this recipe with paprika, a slightly spicy seasoning. Serve it with poached, fried, or scrambled eggs or egg whites.

MAKES 4 SERVINGS

1 tablespoon olive oil

1 teaspoon paprika

½ teaspoon sugar

½ teaspoon salt

2 sweet potatoes (about 1½ pounds), peeled and chopped (about 5 cups)

½ bell pepper, chopped (about ½ cup)

½ sweet onion, chopped (about 1 cup)

1 tablespoon chopped fresh parsley

◉ Preheat the oven to 350°F. Line a rimmed baking sheet with parchment paper. Set aside.

◉ Combine the olive oil, paprika, sugar, and salt in a large bowl and stir until combined. Add the sweet potatoes, bell pepper, and onion, and toss for about a minute, until the ingredients are thoroughly coated with the spice mixture.

⊙ Arrange the vegetables in a single layer on the prepared baking sheet. Cover with aluminum foil and bake for 20 minutes. Carefully remove the foil and poke the sweet potato with a fork to see if it is starting to become tender. Continue roasting, uncovered, for 25 to 30 minutes, until the vegetables are very tender. Scatter the parsley on top just before serving.

Florentine Egg Cups

These are packed with protein and iron (from the spinach). You can make a whole batch and reheat in the microwave as necessary.

MAKES 12 SERVINGS

8 eggs, lightly beaten

1 (16-ounce) package frozen chopped spinach, thawed and squeezed dry (about 1⅓ cups)

¾ cup grated Parmesan cheese

2 tablespoons prepared pesto sauce (optional and check the sodium content)

6 grape tomatoes, halved

⊙ Preheat the oven to 375°F. Place foil muffin liners in a 12-cup muffin pan (if using a silicone muffin pan, which works best for this recipe, you can skip the liners, but make sure to put the pan on a baking sheet before you begin). Set aside.

❂ Combine the eggs, spinach, Parmesan, and pesto sauce in a large bowl and stir until thoroughly combined. Divide the egg mixture among the prepared muffin cups so that each cup is approximately two-thirds full. Place a grape tomato half on top of each cup, cut side up. Bake for 18 to 20 minutes, until a knife inserted in the center of a cup comes out clean.

Main Courses

During Phase 2, your main courses are all about comfort. We've taken the best comfort foods—mac and cheese, meatballs, meat loaf, and much more—and put a heart-healthy spin on all of them. These are true guiltless pleasures that you can feel good about eating.

Vegetarian Chili

We wanted to include a vegetarian option for the non-meat-eaters among you. But this recipe is a big hit even for meat lovers. We make it often. Serve it with a salad and a side of bread.

MAKES 6 SERVINGS (1½ CUPS EACH)

1 onion, finely chopped

3 cloves garlic, minced

1 (4-ounce) can chopped green chiles (do not drain)

1 (14.5-ounce) can diced tomatoes (low sodium)

1 cup corn

½ teaspoon salt-free seasoning blend, such as Mrs. Dash

1 teaspoon dried oregano

I teaspoon ground cumin

I½ tablespoons chili powder

2 (13.5-ounce) cans red kidney beans, rinsed and drained

5 cups low-sodium tomato or vegetable juice

❂ Place the onion and garlic in a large saucepan. Heat over low heat, stirring frequently, until the onions are soft and translucent. Add water as needed to prevent sticking.

❂ Add the rest of the ingredients and stir thoroughly. Cook over medium heat until bubbling. Reduce heat and simmer 20 minutes or longer. May be served over brown rice or pasta as appetite increases.

Old-Fashioned Mac and Cheese

Traditional macaroni and cheese is one of life's greatest comforts, but it's not one of the greatest things for your life. Loaded with fat from milk, butter, and cheese as well as lots of refined starch, it contains nearly everything your doctor has cautioned you not to eat—with the one exception of sugar. You can still enjoy the taste of this creamy dish, though, just by making a few substitutions: whole-grain pasta for the refined version, low-fat cheese for full-fat, and skim milk for whole. This recipe also substitutes Benecol, a margarine shown to reduce cholesterol, for butter.

SERVES 8

2 tablespoons Benecol

2 tablespoons whole-wheat flour

I½ cups skim milk

Salt and pepper

3 cups grated low-fat sharp cheddar cheese

1 (8-ounce) box whole-grain elbow macaroni, cooked and drained

¼ cup unsweetened high-fiber breakfast cereal, such as All-Bran

◉ Preheat the oven to 350°F.

◉ In a large saucepan, melt the Benecol over medium heat. Add the flour and stir until smooth. Add the milk, whisk together, and cook until thickened, about 3 minutes. Add salt and pepper to taste and the cheese, cooking until the cheese melts, about 1 minute. Add the macaroni and stir to combine.

◉ Place the cereal in a food processor or blender and blend until smooth.

◉ Pour the macaroni mixture into a 2-quart casserole dish. Sprinkle the blended cereal on top.

◉ Bake until the topping is brown and the cheese is bubbly, about 20 minutes.

Quick and Easy Fajitas

This is a fast recipe that's easy to make ahead of time. Jamie used to make up a bunch and leave them in the fridge for me to warm and eat whenever I felt that I could. They became a family favorite. Corn tortillas are a much heart-healthier option than flour.

MAKES 8 FAJITAS

1 medium onion, sliced in strips

1 large bell pepper, sliced in strips

1 cup sliced mushrooms

9 ounces precooked chicken strips

1 teaspoon ground cumin

1 teaspoon chili powder

Salt-free seasoning blend, such as Mrs. Dash

8 medium corn tortillas

½ cup fat-free shredded cheddar cheese

🌑 Preheat the oven to 350°F.

🌑 Spray a medium saucepan with cooking spray and heat over medium-high heat. Add the onion and cook for 2 minutes, stirring frequently. Add the pepper and mushrooms and cook until they are soft and the onion is translucent, about 5 minutes. Add the chicken and spices. Stir to combine and heat through. Remove from the heat.

🌑 Place a small amount of the mixture in the center of a corn tortilla. Sprinkle about a tablespoon of cheese on top. Fold in the sides and then the bottom. Place in a baking dish. Repeat with the rest of the tortillas. Bake until tortillas are crispy and slightly brown, about 10 to 15 minutes.

Tuna Melt Sandwich

Yes, you really can make something that's warm, comforting, and delicious from a can.

MAKES 2 SERVINGS

1 (6-ounce) can solid white tuna, drained

1 stalk celery, finely chopped (about 3 tablespoons)

1 small onion, minced (about 1 tablespoon)

½ teaspoon drained capers, chopped

1 tablespoon fat-free mayonnaise

2 slices multigrain bread

2 slices reduced-fat cheddar-flavor slices, such as Smart Balance

2 tomato slices

Freshly ground black pepper

- Preheat the oven to 350°F.

- Combine the tuna, celery, onion, and capers in a small bowl and stir until thoroughly combined. Stir in the mayonnaise until completely incorporated. Divide the mixture between 2 slices of bread and arrange on a baking sheet. Top each bread slice with a cheddar-flavor slice and a tomato slice, and sprinkle with pepper. Bake for 8 to 10 minutes, until the cheese is melted.

Turkey Meat Loaf

Standard meat loaf is rich in heart-clogging saturated fat and sodium. This version simply swaps fatty ground beef for lean turkey breast. In lieu of turkey, you can also use extra-lean ground beef or a mixture of extra-lean ground beef and ground turkey breast. By substituting tomato paste for ketchup, this recipe has significantly less sodium than most meat loaf recipes.

MAKES 6 SERVINGS

½ small onion

1 (8-ounce) package sliced mushrooms

2 tablespoons olive oil

I teaspoon salt-free seasoning blend, such as Mrs. Dash

¼ teaspoon ground black pepper

3 tablespoons tomato paste

I tablespoon honey

I tablespoon cider vinegar

I tablespoon water

¼ teaspoon ground allspice

I egg

2 tablespoons Worcestershire sauce

I½ pounds extra-lean turkey breast

½ cup whole-wheat breadcrumbs or low-sodium panko (Japanese-style breadcrumbs)

◉ Preheat the oven to 375°F. Coat a 4 x 8-inch loaf pan with cooking spray and set aside.

◉ Chop the onion into 3 or 4 pieces and place in the bowl of a food processor, along with the mushrooms. Pulse 4 or 5 times, until finely chopped.

◉ Heat the oil in a large nonstick skillet over medium-high heat. Add the mushroom mixture, salt substitute, and pepper. Cook, stirring occasionally, for about 5 minutes, or until browned. Remove from the heat and allow to cool slightly.

◉ Meanwhile, mix the tomato paste, honey, vinegar, water, and allspice in a small bowl and set aside.

◉ Combine the egg and Worcestershire sauce in a large bowl and beat lightly. Add the mushroom mixture and turkey. Mix with a fork or clean hands until thoroughly combined. Mix in the breadcrumbs and transfer to the prepared loaf pan. Shape into a loaf, pressing down on the sides to form a slight mound in the center. Spread the tomato mixture evenly over the top and sides of the loaf. Bake for 45 minutes, or until a thermometer inserted in the center registers 165°F. Let rest for 10 minutes before slicing. This can also be used as a turkey or lean beef meatball recipe.

Butternut Squash Mac and Cheese

This classic casserole looks a lot like conventional mac and cheese and tastes appropriately creamy, but it actually employs very little dairy. Instead you'll make the sauce from pureed squash and vegetable broth.

MAKES 4 SERVINGS

2 cups multigrain macaroni

1 (12-ounce) package chopped butternut squash (about 3 cups)

¼ cup reduced-sodium vegetable broth

¼ cup fat-free ricotta cheese

5 reduced-fat cheddar-flavor slices, such as Smart Balance

⅛ teaspoon ground nutmeg

½ cup whole-wheat breadcrumbs or low-sodium panko (Japanese-style breadcrumbs)

1 tablespoon olive oil

1 tablespoon Parmesan cheese

❀ Preheat the oven to 350°F. Coat an 8 x 8-inch baking dish with cooking spray. Set aside.

In a large pot, bring 2 quarts of water to a boil, add the macaroni, and cook for 5 minutes, or until al dente. Drain and place in the prepared baking dish.

Meanwhile, place the squash and vegetable broth in a large microwavable bowl. Cover and cook on high for 4 minutes, or until the squash is very tender.

Transfer the squash and cooking liquid to a food processor. Add the ricotta, cheese slices, and nutmeg and process for about 1 minute, until very smooth.

Pour the squash mixture over the macaroni and stir until thoroughly coated.

Toss the breadcrumbs, olive oil, and Parmesan in a small bowl until thoroughly combined. Scatter the mixture over the macaroni and bake for 25 minutes, or until lightly browned.

Maple-Roasted Squash

This is a very basic dish that's great served alongside poultry or pork or all by itself for those with smaller appetites. The winter squash is an excellent source of heart-healthy antioxidants, as well as vitamins B_1 and C, folic acid, pantothenic acid, potassium, and fiber.

MAKES 4 SERVINGS

1 acorn squash

1 tablespoon Benecol

1 tablespoon maple syrup

¼ teaspoon paprika

⅛ teaspoon salt

❀ Preheat the oven to 350°F.

❀ Slice the squash in half lengthwise, scoop out and discard the seeds. Place each half cut-side down and slice crosswise into 4 pieces.

❀ In a large microwave-safe bowl, heat the Benecol in the microwave for 15 seconds at a time until melted. Stir in the maple syrup, paprika, and salt. Add the squash and toss until well coated. Arrange the squash in a 9 × 13-inch baking dish and cover with aluminum foil. Bake for 45 minutes, or until the squash is tender.

Phase 3 Recipes

Welcome to Phase 3 and the rest of your long, healthy life of eating. The recipes in this collection are just as delicious as they are good for you. We've included a number of recipes designed to help you make the most of certain heart-healthy foods that might currently be unfamiliar to you, especially seafood and vegetables.

In this phase, you'll continue to learn how to defat recipes by using low-fat and nonfat ingredients, add good nutrition with herbs and vegetables, and flavor with salt alternatives. As your appetite increases, add a salad or a brothy soup to start. Enjoy!

Seafood Dishes

Seafood ranks as one of the best heart-healthy protein sources around. Nearly all varieties are naturally low in calories and fat, and those that are not (salmon, tuna, herring, anchovies) contain a heart-healthy type of fat called omega-3 fatty acids.

Fish is also simple to prepare. You squeeze some lemon, sprinkle some Mrs. Dash on top, and bake at 450°F until cooked through. The problem with seafood? If you are not used to preparing it, it may take a few times before you get the cooking just right. That's why we've included these recipes to help you get started.

Oven-Baked Salmon Cakes with Cucumber Relish

Fresh wild salmon is great for your heart. But if you are on a tight budget, try this recipe, which uses canned salmon. It's much less expensive but just as healthy. Prepare the salmon cakes ahead of time, freezing them and baking them as needed. The cucumber relish in this recipe is a simple side accompaniment that offers a tasty (and lighter) alternative to old-fashioned tartar sauce.

MAKES 4 SERVINGS

1 cucumber, peeled, seeded, and diced

2 tablespoons cider vinegar

1 teaspoon sugar

½ teaspoon dried dill

1 egg

½ small sweet onion, grated (about ⅓ cup)

2 tablespoons chopped fresh parsley

2 teaspoons salt-free seasoning blend, such as Mrs. Dash

2 teaspoons canola mayonnaise

1 (14.75-ounce) can red salmon, drained

½ cup whole-wheat breadcrumbs or low-sodium panko (Japanese-style breadcrumbs)

2 tablespoons cornmeal

❂ Preheat the oven to 350°F. Coat a small baking sheet with cooking spray and set aside.

❂ To make the cucumber relish, in a small bowl, combine the cucumber, vinegar, sugar, and dill. Cover with ¼ cup water and refrigerate until serving.

❂ In a large bowl, combine the egg, onion, parsley, seasoning, and mayonnaise. Stir with a fork until thoroughly combined. Add the salmon and mix thoroughly. Add the breadcrumbs and stir until thoroughly combined. Shape the mixture into 4 patties and dredge in cornmeal (see Note). Arrange on the prepared baking sheet and bake for 20 minutes, or until lightly browned. Serve with the cucumber relish.

Note: These patties freeze exceptionally well and can be made ahead and baked later. Simply adjust the baking time to 25 minutes.

Roasted Shrimp and Broccoli

This delicious combination is low on effort because you just roast it in the oven, requiring only one pan and just a few minutes prep time. It's lightly seasoned with cumin and garlic, and a fresh squeeze of lemon at the end makes this dish sing.

2 tablespoons olive oil

½ teaspoon salt

½ teaspoon freshly ground black pepper

I tablespoon minced garlic

I teaspoon ground cumin

I pound large shrimp, peeled and deveined

2 bunches broccoli (about I pound)

½ lemon, juiced

❂ Preheat the oven to 425°F.

❂ Mix I tablespoon of the olive oil, ¼ teaspoon of the salt, ¼ teaspoon of the pepper, the garlic, and the cumin in a large bowl. Add the shrimp and toss to coat. Refrigerate while preparing the broccoli.

❂ Cut the broccoli into walnut-size florets (approximately 5 cups). Mix the remaining I tablespoon olive oil, ¼ teaspoon salt, and ¼ teaspoon pepper in a separate bowl and add the broccoli. Toss well and spread on a rimmed baking sheet. Roast for 7 to 10 minutes, or until bright green.

❂ Spread the shrimp on the same baking sheet and bake for 5 minutes longer, until the shrimp are pink. Toss the broccoli and shrimp together with the lemon juice and serve.

Poultry Dishes

Like fish, poultry is a great low-fat protein option. Most of the fat in a bird is located in and just under the skin. As long as you remove the skin (or buy any number of skinless options), you'll have a filling, low-fat source of sustenance.

To save money, buy chicken in bulk, freezing it in recipe-size portions (4 pieces or 1 pound to a bag). The morning before you wish to prepare a recipe, remove your chicken from the freezer and place it in the refrigerator so it can defrost during the day.

The following recipes will give you plenty of quick and easy ways to prepare this heart-healthy food so you never have the thought, "Chicken again?!"

Oven-"Fried" Chicken Fingers with Apricot Curry Dipping Sauce

This dish offers the same satisfying, crunchy texture of fried chicken— without, of course, all the fat. Soaked in buttermilk and coated with Japanese breadcrumbs (and perhaps a little ground flaxseed), these are served with a light dipping sauce that's a lower-sodium alternative to barbecue sauce.

MAKES 4 SERVINGS

⅓ cup buttermilk

¼ teaspoon salt

¼ teaspoon freshly ground black pepper

1 pound chicken tenders

1½ cups Multi-Bran Chex cereal

¾ cup whole-wheat breadcrumbs or low-sodium panko
   (Japanese-style breadcrumbs)

2 tablespoons sesame seeds

¼ cup all-fruit apricot spread

½ teaspoon fresh lemon juice

¼ teaspoon curry powder

¼ teaspoon grated ginger

◉ Preheat oven to 350°F. Coat a rimmed baking sheet with cooking spray.

◉ Combine the buttermilk, salt, and pepper in a large bowl. Add the chicken and toss to coat. Set aside.

◉ Place the cereal in a zip-top bag and crush gently with the bottom of a jar to form crumbs. Transfer to a large bowl and add the breadcrumbs and sesame seeds.

◉ Dredge the chicken pieces in the crumb mixture, pressing as needed to ensure an even coating, and arrange on the prepared sheet. Bake for 15 minutes, or until cooked through.

◉ While the chicken is in the oven, prepare the sauce by placing the apricot spread, lemon juice, curry powder, and ginger in a small microwave-safe bowl. Microwave the apricot mixture on high for 30 to 45 seconds, until warmed through. Stir well to make sure the ingredients are thoroughly combined, and keep warm until ready to serve.

Turkey Meatballs

Nothing says comfort like spaghetti and meatballs. But unlike traditional recipes, these are made with walnuts in place of some of the breadcrumbs. This helps cut down on the sodium as well as adding heart-healthy monounsaturated fats. Also, these are oven-baked, so there's no need to stand in front of a hot stove while they cook. Just like mama would have made if she'd known better.

MAKES 6 SERVINGS

FOR THE MEATBALLS

- 2 teaspoons olive oil
- ½ cup walnuts
- ½ onion, coarsely chopped
- 1½ pounds extra-lean ground turkey
- 1 egg, lightly beaten
- 1 tablespoon minced garlic
- 1 heaping teaspoon dried oregano
- ½ cup nonfat milk
- ¼ cup grated Parmesan cheese
- ½ cup whole-wheat breadcrumbs or low-sodium panko (Japanese-style breadcrumbs)

FOR THE SPAGHETTI AND SAUCE

- 1 (28-ounce) can no-salt-added crushed tomatoes
- 2 tablespoons olive oil
- ½ onion, chopped
- 1 tablespoon tomato paste
- 12 ounces multigrain spaghetti
- Basil, for garnish

TO MAKE THE MEATBALLS: Preheat the oven to 350°F. Coat a rimmed baking sheet with olive oil and set aside.

Pulse the walnuts and onion in a food processor until very finely chopped. Transfer to a large bowl. Add the turkey, egg, garlic, oregano, and milk. Mix well with a fork until thoroughly combined. Add the Parmesan and breadcrumbs and mix well. Form into tablespoon-size meatballs and arrange on the prepared baking sheet (a small cookie scoop works especially well for this task).

❀ Bake for about 10 to 15 minutes, until cooked through. Transfer to the sauce and cook 20 minutes longer.

TO MAKE THE SAUCE: While the meatballs are in the oven, combine the tomatoes, olive oil, onion, and tomato paste in a 3½-quart pot. Bring to a simmer and transfer the meatballs to the pot when they are finished baking. Let simmer 20 minutes longer while you prepare the pasta.

❀ Bring a large pot of water to a boil and cook the pasta according to the instructions on the box until slightly firm to the bite. Drain the pasta and toss lightly in the sauce and meatballs. Garnish with basil for added color.

Desserts

My motto is "Eat to Live" most of the time. For the rest of the time: there's dessert! You need a little culinary joy in life to keep your spirits up and, during the initial weeks after surgery, sometimes something sweet is the only thing you can stomach at all.

If possible, try to satisfy an urge for something sweet with something healthy, such as fresh fruit topped with a small amount of nonfat whipped cream.

If your urge for sweetness is more extreme, then try one of the following delicious desserts. Now here's the surprising news about dessert: It doesn't have to be bad for your heart! The following desserts are just as good for your health as they are for your taste buds. Talk about a guiltless pleasure!

To make over your own personal recipes, try substituting whole-grain flour for refined flour. Add fruit and nuts if possible. And substitute applesauce or pureed prunes for up to half the butter in a recipe (1 tablespoon of sauce for every 1 tablespoon of butter).

Heart-Smart Peanut Butter Balls

Don't waste a molecule of guilt on these little bite-size treats. A variation on a no-bake cookie, these treats offer omega-3-fortified peanut butter, calcium-rich powdered milk, fiber-rich cereal, and a little honey.

MAKES 4 SERVINGS (2 BALLS EACH)

½ cup caramel-flavored high-fiber cereal, such as Fiber One

¼ cup creamy peanut or soy nut butter, preferably omega-3-enriched

2 tablespoons honey

2 tablespoons nonfat dried milk

◉ Place the cereal in a zip-top bag and crush gently with the bottom of a jar to form crumbs. Set aside.

◉ Combine the peanut butter and honey in a small bowl and stir until smooth. Add the milk and cereal and mash with the back of a fork until thoroughly combined. Divide the mixture into 8 equal pieces and shape into balls. Refrigerate until chilled. Then enjoy.

Nutty Natural Chocolate Spread

For all you Nutella fans out there, this is a much healthier alternative that draws on omega-3-enriched peanut butter, 75% dark chocolate, and a little honey. There are plenty of ways to enjoy this spread. Pair it with fresh fruit or a little bread.

MAKES 2 SERVINGS

- 1 ounce 75% dark chocolate, coarsely chopped
- 1 tablespoon creamy peanut butter, preferably omega-3-enriched
- 1 teaspoon honey
- 1 to 2 drops almond extract

Place the chocolate and peanut butter in a small microwave-safe bowl and microwave on high for 30 to 45 seconds, until the chocolate is softened and beginning to melt. Stir until the chocolate is completely melted. Stir in the honey and almond extract.

Serve warm as a dip for strawberries, pineapple, and bananas, or let cool 20 minutes, until the chocolate assumes a spreadable consistency, and then slather on fresh fruit or toasted bread.

Strawberries and Cream

Fat-free cream? Yes, it's true. By mixing together cottage cheese with a little buttermilk, you end up with a sweet, creamy cheese that tastes delicious.

½ cup low-fat cottage cheese

1 tablespoon buttermilk

¾ teaspoon fresh lemon juice

1½ teaspoons brown sugar

1 cup strawberries, rinsed, hulled, and quartered

❁ Puree the cottage cheese, buttermilk, and lemon juice in a blender until smooth. Add the brown sugar. Mix.

❁ Top the strawberries with the cheese mixture and chill before serving.

13

The Back-to-Life Resources

IN THE FOLLOWING PAGES, WE'VE SUGGESTED A FEW HELPFUL RE-
sources to help you in your quest to reclaim the next chapter of your life.
You'll find contact information for support groups, services, heart-disease-
themed charity events, and much more. You'll find a list of my favorite and
funniest books and films. And you'll find an assortment of training plans that
will help you train for walking, running, cycling, and swimming events.

Report Cards

To learn about a physician's or hospital's track record, use any of the following hospital report-card services. Check our website at www.backtolifethe
book.com for additional resources.

America's Best Hospitals
U.S. News & World Report
www.health.usnews.com/health/best-hospitals

Guide to Hospitals
Consumers' Checkbook
www.checkbook.org

Health Care Choices
www.healthcarechoices.org

HealthGrades Inc.
www.healthgrades.com

The LeapFrog Group
www.leapfroggroup.org

Quality Check

The Joint Commission on Accreditation of Health Care Organizations
www.jcaho.org

Inspiring Books and Audio Series

I read and used the following books after my diagnosis. I hope you find
them as helpful as I did.

The Art of Happiness, by the Dalai Lama and Howard Cutler, M.D.
The Complete Idiot's Guide to a Happy, Healthy Heart,
  by Deborah S. Romaine

The Complete Idiot's Guide to Managing Stress, by Jeff Davidson

It's Not About the Bike, by Lance Armstrong

Learn to Relax, by Mike George

Minding the Body, Mending the Mind, by Joan Borysenko

Funny Movies

In addition to my Jackie Mason DVDs, funny movies helped me keep things in perspective, and use the power of laughter to ease depression and stress. Below is a listing of some of the funniest movies of all time.

Ace Ventura: Pet Detective

Airplane

Animal House

Arthur

Beverly Hills Cop

Big

Bill and Ted's Excellent Adventure

Blazing Saddles

Caddyshack

Dumb & Dumber

Fast Times at Ridgemont High

The Jerk

M*A*S*H

Meet the Fockers

The Naked Gun

Napoleon Dynamite

Old School

The Producers

Shrek

South Park: Bigger, Longer & Uncut

Stripes

There's Something About Mary

Wedding Crashers

The Wedding Singer

Support Groups and Support Resources

Survivor support groups can help you feel less alone. Look for one in your area. You can find out more about local groups through your local hospital or your cardiac rehabilitation program. Here are a few organizations to try.

Cardiac Rehabilitation

The American Association of Cardiovascular and Pulmonary Rehabilitation

www.aacvpr.org

At this site you can search for a program near you.

CarePages

www.carepages.com

Use this site to more easily keep others up to date on your heath status.

Mended Hearts

www.mendedhearts.org

A national volunteer support group for heart patients and their loved ones.

American Heart Association

1-800-AHA-USA-1

www.americanheart.org

Your local chapter might also be able to help you find a support group near you.

Women Heart Community

www.womenheart.org

An online support group for women with heart disease.

Heart2Hearts

www.heart2hearts.co.uk

An online support group for people with heart disease.

Charity Events

Raising money for a charity can help add meaning to whatever challenge you decide to take on. Here are a few heart-disease-related charities. We've included some that benefit diabetes, as the two diseases are often connected.

StepOut Walk to Fight Diabetes

American Diabetes Association (ADA)

(888) DIABETES (342-2383)

www.stepout.diabetes.org

Funds generated from this walkathon, which is held in different locations throughout the United States, go toward the ADA's research, education, and advocacy programs.

Start! Heart Walk

American Heart Association (AHA)

(800) AHA-USA-1 (242-8721)

www.americanheart.org/start

The Start! Heart Walk promotes physical activity while raising funds for saving lives from heart disease and stroke, two potential complications of diabetes.

Walk to Cure Diabetes

Juvenile Diabetes Research Foundation (JDRF) International

(888) 533-WALK (9255)

www.walk.jdrf.org

The JDRF International organizes walks throughout the year to raise funds for type-1 diabetes research.

The Back-to-Life Training Plans

In the following pages, you'll find training advice and plans for common challenges, including running, cycling, and swimming events. Check our website at www.backtolifethebook.com for updates on other physical activities and challenges.

Training Plans for Walking, Jogging, and Running Challenges

You can use the following plans to complete the corresponding distances at any pace—whether you plan to walk, run, or do a combination of both. When training for walking and running distances, use a soft surface whenever possible. Walking and especially running can inflict a lot of impact on the body. The softer your running surface, the less impact your joints absorb. Try to do at least some of your training on a dirt trail or grass if possible.

Also, for your first attempt after surgery, you probably should either walk the entire distance if you are a beginning exerciser, or do a combination of walking and running if you are a former runner.

If you plan to advance to running, start your training by running for 1 minute per every 5 minutes of walking. Slowly increase your running time—adding no more than a minute a week—until you are running for 5 minutes for every 5 minutes of walking. At that point you can either stick with the 5-and-5 approach, or you can slowly decrease your walking time until you are walking 1 minute out of every 5 to 10 running minutes, or one minute after every mile.

R = Rest, and rest means no weight-bearing exercise. It's okay to do light cross-training on your rest days (a mild walk, swimming, cycling), but do not run.

Numbers = miles, not kilometers.

5K (3.1 MILES)

This plan takes you from beginner to race ready. There's no base required.

Week	M	T	W	Th	F	S	S
1	R	1 mile	R	1 mile	R	1 mile	R
2	R	1	R	1	R	1.5	R
3	R	1	R	1	R	2	R
4	R	1.5	R	1	R	2	R
5	R	2	R	2	R	2.5	R
6	R	2.5	R	2.5	R	3	R
7	R	2.5	R	2.5	R	3	R
8	R	2	R	2	R	5K race	R

10K (6.2 MILES)

You should be able to comfortably run or walk 10 miles a week, 3 miles at a time, before attempting the 10K. It's a great idea to finish a 5K first. Doing so will get you used to racing—especially the masses of people—before your big day. During your sessions, just put one foot in front of the other. Don't worry about speed. For now, your goal is to finish. You can work on finishing in record time in subsequent races.

R = Rest, and rest means no weight-bearing exercise. It's okay to do light cross-training on your rest days (a mild walk, swimming, cycling), but do not run.

Numbers = miles, not kilometers.

Week	M	T	W	Th	F	S	S
1	R	3 miles	R	3 miles	R	3 miles	R
2	R	3	R	R	R	4	R
3	R	3	R	3	R	5	R
4	R	3	R	3	R	6	R
5	R	3	R	3	R	7	R
6	R	3	R	3	R	7	R
7	R	3	R	3	R	5	R
8	R	3	R	3	R	10K race	R

HALF MARATHON (13.1 MILES)

If you plan to one day complete a marathon, the half is the ideal marathon prep race. On its own, the half is a great race to prove to yourself that you are truly alive. Tackle this plan only once you've increased your fitness to running or walking at least 5 miles in one stretch and are averaging about 15 miles a week.

On this plan, you'll train three days a week, increasing both your base mileage and the miles completed during your longest session. Note that this plan assumes you have the bulk of your free time on the weekends. If you have a different schedule, alter the plan as needed so you are doing your longest sessions on the days you have the most time. During your final two weeks you will taper your mileage, running or walking less than you did in previous weeks. This will allow your body to rest and recover for your big day. You'll also notice that here and there in the schedule, there's an easy week, when I suggest you cut back some on your mileage. Again, these are designed to help your body (not to mention mind) repair itself so it's ready for the weeks to come.

R = Rest, and rest means no weight-bearing exercise. It's okay to do light cross-training on your rest days (a mild walk, swimming, cycling), but do not run.

Numbers = miles, not kilometers.

Week	M	T	W	Th	F	S	S
1	R	4 miles	R	4 miles	R	5 miles	R
2	R	4	R	4	R	6	R
3	R	4	R	4	R	7	R
4	R	5	R	5	R	8	R
5	R	5	R	5	R	5	R
6	R	5	R	5	R	8	R
7	R	5	R	5	R	10	R
8	R	5	R	5	R	12	R
9	R	4	R	4	R	5	R
10	R	3	R	3	R	half marathon	R

MARATHON (26.2 MILES)

Tackle this plan only after you've finished one of the shorter race distances and you can comfortably run or walk 5 miles and are regularly completing 15 to 20 weekly miles. On this plan, you'll train three to four days a week, increasing your base mileage from 15 to 20 miles to more than 30 weekly miles. The plan will very gradually increase both your weekly miles and the miles completed during your longest session. Note that this plan assumes you have the bulk of your free time on the weekends. If you have a different schedule, alter the plan as needed so you are doing your longest sessions on the days you have the most time. During your final two weeks you will taper your mileage, running or walking less than you did in previous weeks. This will allow your body to rest and recover for your big day. You'll also notice that here and there in the schedule, there's an easy week, when I suggest you cut back some on your mileage. Again, these are designed to help your body (not to mention mind) repair itself so it's ready for the weeks to come.

R = Rest, and rest means no weight-bearing exercise. It's okay to do light cross-training on your rest days (a mild walk, swimming, cycling), but do not run.

Numbers = miles, not kilometers.

Week	M	T	W	Th	F	S	S
1	R	4 miles	R	4 miles	R	5 miles	3 miles
2	R	4	R	4	R	6	3
3	R	4	R	5	R	7	3
4	R	4	R	6	R	8	R
5	R	5	R	6	R	9	R
6	R	5	R	6	R	6	R
7	R	5	R	6	R	10	R
8	R	5	R	6	R	10	R
9	R	5	R	6	R	12	R
10	R	5	R	6	R	14	R
11	R	5	R	6	R	6	R
12	R	5	R	6	R	16	R
13	R	6	R	6	R	16	R
14	R	6	R	6	R	18	R
15	R	6	R	6	R	20	R
16	R	5	R	5	R	10	R
17	R	3	R	3	R	5	R
18	R	3	R	3	R	marathon	R

Training Plans for Cycling Challenges

If you are a cyclist, you have plenty of fun and motivating rides to choose from. Where I live, there's the 42-mile Five Boro Bike Tour. The trek goes though five boroughs traffic free, taking you over the Queensboro Bridge, the Pulaski Bridge, and the Verrazano-Narrows Bridge. You'll even ride on the FDR Drive, which is usually closed to cyclists.

If you are feeling more adventurous, you can do a Century (100 miles) or even a multiday ride, such as The Register's Annual Great Bicycle Ride Across Iowa (RAGBRAI), which is a weeklong 442-mile route across southern Iowa.

Below you'll find training plans for three common ride distances: 25 miles, 50 miles, and 100 miles. Use the plan that corresponds most closely to your chosen ride distance. For instance, if you are doing a 40-mile ride, use the 50-mile plan. Use this advice no matter which plan you are using:

Ride with others. This reduces anxiety, which can include worrying about being stranded with a flat or about going out too far and not being able to make it back. Your ride group can draft you (by riding in front of you and breaking the wind) to make a training ride go a little easier. A riding buddy can also place a hand on your back and push you forward a bit to help you overcome difficulty on a hill.

Ride at a pace somewhere between 6 and 15 miles per hour. Most official rides have safety and technical help as long as you can hold this pace. Try to keep your pace consistent during your rides.

If you are a beginner, start off with a coach, training club, or experienced rider. You'll need someone who can walk you through the initial learning curve of choosing a bike and other equipment, learning basic handling skills (such as the art of riding in traffic), and navigating routes without getting lost.

25-MILE TRAINING PLAN

This plan takes you from beginner to ride ready.

R = Rest, and rest means no weight-bearing exercise. It's okay to do light cross-training on your rest days.

Numbers = miles, not kilometers.

Week	M	T	W	Th	F	S	S
1	R	5 miles	R	5 miles	R	5 miles	5 miles
2	R	5	R	5	R	5	5
3	R	5	R	5	R	10	5
4	R	10	R	10	R	10	10
5	R	10	R	10	R	15	10
6	R	10	R	10	R	15	10
7	R	15	R	15	R	20	15
8	R	15	R	15	R	25	15

50-MILE TRAINING PLAN

You should be able to comfortably ride 15 miles before attempting this plan. This plan assumes that you work during the week and have a limited amount of time to devote to the bike. You can ride more than the plan calls for. This is a minimum.

R = Rest, and rest means no weight-bearing exercise. It's okay to do light cross-training on your rest days.

Numbers = miles, not kilometers.

Week	M	T	W	Th	F	S	S
1	R	10 miles	R	10 miles	R	15 miles	10 miles
2	R	10	R	10	R	20	10
3	R	15	R	15	R	25	15
4	R	15	R	15	R	30	15
5	R	15	R	15	R	35	15
6	R	15	R	15	R	40	15
7	R	15	R	15	R	45	15
8	R	20	R	20	R	50	20

Century (100-Mile) Training Plan

You should be able to comfortably ride 30 miles before attempting this plan. This plan assumes that you work during the week and have a limited amount of time to devote to the bike. You can ride more than the plan calls for. This is a minimum.

R = Rest, and rest means no weight-bearing exercise. It's okay to do light cross-training on your rest days.

Numbers = miles, not kilometers.

Week	M	T	W	Th	F	S	S
1	R	15 miles	R	15 miles	R	30 miles	15 miles
2	R	15	R	15	R	35	15
3	R	15	R	15	R	40	15
4	R	15	R	15	R	45	15
5	R	20	R	20	R	50	20
6	R	20	R	20	R	55	20
7	R	25	R	25	R	60	25
8	R	20	R	20	R	65	20
9	R	20	R	20	R	71	20
10	R	20	R	20	R	75	20
11	R	20	R	20	R	85	20
12	R	20	R	20	R	100	20

Training Plans for Swimming Challenges

If you are doing any other form of exercise (weights, walking, cycling), you probably can get away with just two swims a week. You can do more (up to five swims a week), but don't do less.

The best strategy is to start wherever you are comfortable, even if it's just one or two lengths, and slowly build from there. Time your workouts, increasing your total session time by about 10 minutes each week. Let's say you start with 1 length and it takes you a few minutes to swim it. Then increase your distance by 1 to 4 pool lengths a week (10 swimming minutes at a time) until you can swim the number of lengths you need to swim for any given distance.

If you have little swimming experience, start with a coach. You'll be confronting two different fears—the fear of exertion and the fear of not being able to get enough air (because your face is in the water part of the time). A coach can help keep you calm.

Here's how many lengths you need to swim for some popular swim distances:

Quarter mile: This is about 500 yards, which translates to 20 lengths in a 25-yard pool and 8 lengths in a 50-meter pool.

Half mile: 32 lengths in a 25-yard pool or 16 lengths in a 50-meter pool

1.5K (1 mile): 68 lengths in a 25-yard pool or 30 lengths in a 50-meter pool

1.2 miles: 80 lengths in a 25-yard pool or 40 lengths in a 50-meter pool

Please stay in touch!

We'd love to hear from you. Please visit us at www.backtolifethebook .com. Let us know how your cardiac comeback is going. Have you become Unbeatable? Please tell us all about it! Would you like more advice? Please ask. We continually update the site and try to make it as useful as possible. We look forward to hearing about the next chapter of your life.

Notes

Chapter 3

1. Simpson T, Lee ER, "Individual factors that influence sleep after cardiac surgery," *American Journal of Critical Care* May 1996 5 (3) 182–189.

2. Redeker NS, Ruggiero JS, Hedges C, "Sleep is related to physical function and emotional well-being after cardiac surgery," *Nursing Research* May 2004 53 (3) 154–162.

3. Taylor DJ, Mallory LJ, Lichstein KL, Durrence HH, Riedel BW, Bush AJ, "Comorbidity of chronic insomnia with medical problems," *Sleep* Feb. 2007 30 (2) 213–218.

4. Kanda K, Tochihara Y, Ohnaka T, "Bathing before sleep in the young and in the elderly," *European Journal of Applied Physiology and Occupational Physiology* July 1999 80(2):71–75.

5. Dorsey CM, Teicher MH, Cohen-Zion M, Stefanovic L, Satlin A, Tartarini W, Harper D, Lukas SE, "Core body temperature and sleep of older female insomniacs before and after passive body heating," *Sleep* Nov. 1999 22(7):891–898.

6. Barker SB, Knisely JS, McCain NL, Best AM, "Measuring stress and immune response in healthcare and professionals following interaction with a therapy dog: a pilot study," *Psychological Reports* June 2005 96 (3 Pt 1) 713–729.

Chapter 4

1. Porter J, Jick H, "Addiction rare in patients treated with narcotics," *New England Journal of Medicine* Jan 10 1980;302(2):123.

2. Sendelbach SE, Halm MA, Doran KA, Miller EH, Gaillard P, "Effects of music therapy on physiological and psychological outcomes for patients undergoing cardiac surgery," *Journal of Cardiovascular Nursing* May–Jun 2006;21(3):194–200.

3. Krout RE, "The effects of single-session music therapy interventions on the observed and self-reported levels of pain control, physical comfort, and relaxation of hospice patients," *American Journal of Hospital Palliative Care* Nov–Dec 2001;18(6):383–390.

4. Voss JA, Good M, Yates B, Baun MM, Thompson A, Hertzog M, "Sedative music reduces anxiety and pain during chair rest after open-heart surgery," *Pain* Nov 2004;112(1–2):197–203.

5. Twiss E, Seaver J, McCaffrey R, "The effect of music listening on older adults undergoing cardiovascular surgery," *Nursing in Critical Care* Sep–Oct 2006;11(5):224–231.

6. Kukuk P, Lungenhausen M, Molsberger A, Endres HG, "Long-term improvement in pain coping for cLBP and gonarthrosis patients following body

needle acupuncture: a prospective cohort study," *European Journal of Medicine Research* Jun 22, 2005;10(6):263–272.

7. Haake M, Müller HH, Schade-Brittinger C, Basler HD, Schäfer H, Maier C, Endres HG, Trampisch HJ, Molsberger A, "German Acupuncture Trials (GERAC) for chronic low back pain: randomized, multicenter, blinded, parallel-group trial with 3 groups," *Archives of Internal Medicine* Sep 24 2007;167(17):1892–1898.

8. Curiati JA, Bocchi E, Freire JO, Arantes AC, Braga M, Garcia Y, Guimarães G, Fo WJ, "Meditation reduces sympathetic activation and improves the quality of life in elderly patients with optimally treated heart failure: a prospective randomized study," *Journal of Alternative and Complementary Med* Jun 2005;11(3):465–472.

9. Ashton RC Jr, Whitworth GC, Seldomridge JA, Shapiro PA, Michler RE, Smith CR, Rose EA, Fisher S, Oz MC, "The effects of self-hypnosis on quality of life following coronary artery bypass surgery: preliminary results of a prospective, randomized trial," *Journal of Alternative and Complementary Medicine* Fall 1995;1(3):285–290.

10. Ashton C Jr, Whitworth GC, Seldomridge JA, Shapiro PA, Weinberg AD, Michler RE, Smith CR, Rose EA, Fisher S, Oz MC, "Self-hypnosis reduces anxiety following coronary artery bypass surgery. A prospective, randomized trial," *Journal of Cardiovascular Surgery* (Torino). Feb 1997;38(1):69–75.

11. De Pascalis V, Cacace I, Massicolle F, "Focused analgesia in waking and hypnosis: effects on pain, memory, and somatosensory event-related potentials," *Pain* Jan 2008;134(1-2):197–208. Epub Nov 26, 2007.

12. Holland B, Pokorny ME, "Slow stroke back massage: its effect on patients in a rehabilitation setting," *Rehabilitation Nursing* Sep–Oct 2001;26(5):182–186.

13. Kutner JS, Smith MC, Corbin L, Hemphill L, Benton K, Mellis BK, Beaty B, Felton S, Yamashita TE, Bryant LL, Fairclough DL, "Massage therapy versus

simple touch to improve pain and mood in patients with advanced cancer: a randomized trial," *Internal Medicine* Sep 16 2008;149(6):369–379.

14. Seers K, Crichton N, Martin J, Coulson K, Carroll D, "A randomized controlled trial to assess the effectiveness of a single session of nurse administered massage for short term relief of chronic non-malignant pain," *BMC Nursing* Jul 4, 2008;7:10.

15. Moss M, Cook J, Wesnes K, Duckett P, "Aromas of rosemary and lavender essential oils differentially affect cognition and mood in healthy adults," *International Journal of Neuroscience* Jan 2003;113(1):15–38.

16. Kim JT, Wajda M, Cuff G, Serota D, Schlame M, Axelrod DM, Guth AA, Bekker AY, "Evaluation of aromatherapy in treating postoperative pain: pilot study," *Pain Practice* Dec 2006;6(4):273–277.

17. Motomura N, Sakurai A, Yotsuya Y, "Reduction of mental stress with lavender odorant," *Perceptual and Motor Skills* Dec 2001;93(3):713–718.

18. Mahony DL, Burroughs WJ, Hieatt AC, "The effects of laughter on discomfort thresholds: does expectation become reality?" *Journal of General Psychology* Apr 2001;128(2):217–226.

Chapter 5

1. Wennberg P, Lindahl B, Hallmans G, Messner T, Weinehall L, Johansson L, Boman K, Jansson JH, "The effects of commuting activity and occupational and leisure time physical activity on risk of myocardial infarction," *European Journal of Cardiovascular Prevention and Rehabilitation* Dec 2006;13(6):924–930.

2. Peters A, von Klot S, Heier M, Trentinaglia I, Hörmann A, Wichmann HE, Löwel H, "Exposure to traffic and the onset of myocardial infarction," *New England Journal of Medicine* Oct 21, 2004;351(17):1721–1730.

3. Ahlgren E, Lundqvist A, Nordlund A, Aren C, Rutberg H, "Neurocognitive impairment and driving performance after coronary artery bypass surgery," *European Journal of Cardiothoracic Surgery* Mar 2003;23(3):334–340.

4. Shephard RJ, "The acceptable risk of driving after myocardial infarction: are bus drivers a special case?" *Journal of Cardiopulmonary Rehabilitation* May–Jun 1998;18(3):199–208.

5. Wang CC, Kosinski CJ, Schwartzberg JG, Shanklin AV, "Physician's Guide to Assessing and Counseling Older Drivers," Washington, DC: National Highway Traffic Safety Administration; 2003.

Chapter 6

1. Williams AJ, Ross WR, Hutchison S, "Five-year follow-up findings from a randomized controlled trial of cardiac rehabilitation for heart failure," *European Journal of Cardiovascular Prevention and Rehabilitation* April 2008 15 (2) 162–167.

2. Yoshida M, Sato T, Yoshida T, Kohzuki M, "Physical and psychological improvements after phase 11 cardiac rehabilitation in patients with myocardial infarction," *Nursing and Health Sciences* Sep 1, 1999 (3) 163–170.

Chapter 7

1. Ebrahim S, May M, Ben Shlomo Y, McCarron P, Frankel S, Yarnell J, Davey Smith G, "Sexual intercourse and risk of ischaemic stroke and coronary heart disease: the Caerphilly study," *Journal of Epidemiology and Community Health* Feb 2002;56(2):99–102.

2. DeBusk RF, "Evaluating the cardiovascular tolerance for sex," *American Journal of Cardiology* Jul 20, 2000;86(2A):51F–56F.

3. Xue-Rui T, Ying L, Da-Zhong Y, Xiao-Jun C, "Changes of blood pressure and

heart rate during sexual activity in healthy adults," *Blood Pressure Monitoring* Aug 2008;13(4):211–217.

4. Stein RA, "Cardiovascular response to sexual activity," *American Journal of Cardiology* Jul 20, 2000;86(2A):27F–29F.

Chapter 8

1. Saremi A, Arora R, "The Utility of Omega-3 Fatty Acids in Cardiovascular Disease," *American Journal of Therapy* Dec 15, 2008. [Epub ahead of print]

2. Nikolic M, Nikic D, Petrovic B, "Fruit and vegetable intake and the risk for developing coronary heart disease," *Central European Journal of Public Health* 2008 16 (1) 17–20.

3. Mellen PB, Walsh TF, Herrington DM, "Whole grain intake and cardiovascular disease: a meta-analysis," *Nutrition, Metabolism & Cardiovascular Diseases* 2008 18 293–290.

4. Law M., "Plant sterol and stanol margarines and health," *British Medical Journal* March 25, 2000; 320(7238): 861–864.

5. Lichtenstein AH, et al, "Diet and lifestyle recommendations revision 2006: a scientific statement from the American Heart Association Nutrition Committee," *Circulation* 2006;114:82–96.

6. Albert CM et al, "Effect of folic acid and B vitamins on risk of cardiovascular events and total mortality among women at high risk for cardiovascular disease: A randomized trial," *Journal of the American Medical Association* May 7, 2008; 299:2027.

7. Block G, Jensen CD, Dalvi TB, Norkus EP, Hudes M, Crawford PB, Holland N, Fung EB, Schumacher L, Harmatz P, "Vitamin C treatment reduces elevated C-reactive protein," *Free Radical Biology and Medicine* Jan 1, 2009;46(1):70–77. Epub Oct 10, 2008.

8. Osganian SK, Stampfer MJ, Rimm E, Spiegelman D, Hu FB, Manson JE, Willett

depression and, 66–68
during sex, 129–30
during sleep, 43–44
multiple experiences of, 125–27
preferences, 38–40
surgery mortality rates, 25, 27
deep breathing
control of panic attack, 118
relaxing effect of, 52, 72, 110, 201
stimulation of appetite, 142
denial, 6–7, 11–14, 37, 70, 146
dental problems, 64
depression
death risk, 66–68
effect on appetite, 140
management strategies, 70–78
painkiller overuse, 60
physical chill from, 53
sexual problems from, 134–35
sleep medications and, 46, 47
symptoms, 68
desserts
Heart-Smart Peanut Butter Balls, 275
Nutty Natural Chocolate Spread, 276
in Phase 2 eating, 145
Strawberries and Cream, 276–77
diet. *See* food and eating
diphenhydramine (Benadryl, Nytol, Sominex), 45
doctor, consultation with
before exercise program, 211, 217
before return to work, 185
calling as needed, 104–6
fear of, 103–4
first postoperative checkup, 104, 106–12
follow-up testing, 90, 113–19
list of questions, 107–8
multiple opinions, 23, 24–25
for problems during or after exercise, 211
for sexual concerns, 130–32
doctors
cardiologists versus cardiac surgeons, 105
changing, 122–25
choosing, 27, 278–79
Doral, 46
doxylamine (Unisom), 45
driving, 95–98

eating. *See* food and eating
echocardiogram, 55, 90, 114
egg(s)
Chinese Egg Drop Soup, 254
Florentine Egg Cups, 258–59
yolks, 156–57
electrocardiogram (EKG), 114–15
emotional pain. *See also* depression
changed self-perception, 17–18
decision to overcome, 20
failure to recover from, 66
following surgery, 18–19
post-traumatic stress disorder, 66–67
typical experiences, 36–39
exercise. *See also* cardiac rehabilitation; outdoor excursions; physical challenge
benefits of, 209–10
blood pressure and, 217
cardiovascular, 210, 212–16
consultation with doctor concerning, 211, 217
medication and, 212
problems during or after, 211
strength training, 210–11, 216–22
stretching, 211, 222–23
types of, 210–11
during workday, 196–97

Fajitas, Quick and Easy, 261–62
fats, dietary, 156–57, 158–59
fear. *See* emotional pain; sleep problems
Fellow of the American College of Surgeons (FACS), 27
fish
in heart-healthy diet, 147–48
Oven-Baked Salmon Cakes with Cucumber Relish, 268–69
Tuna Melt Sandwich, 262–63
fish oil supplements, 147, 174–75
fitness. *See* cardiac rehabilitation; exercise
Florentine Egg Cups, 258–59
food and eating. *See also* Phase 1 recipes; Phase 2 recipes; Phase 3 recipes
balanced meals, 160
food groups and servings, 161
foods to avoid, 153–59
frequent small meals, 142, 144, 160, 202
grocery lists, 162–64
heart-healthy foods, 147–53

sterol-fortified foods, 153
StopAfib.org support group, 199
Strawberries and Cream, 276–77
Strawberry Banana Smoothie, 250–51
strength training, 210–11, 216–22
stress
    job-related, 187–93, 195–204
    physical effects of, 188–89
stress test, 113–14
stretching exercises, 211, 222–23
sugar consumption, 155–56
supplements, 172–78
support
    groups and resources, 72, 81, 216, 246,
        281–82
    pets, 51, 76–77, 99
    support team and advocate, 27–28, 30–32
    true friends, 78–83
    in workplace, 201
surgeon. *See* doctors
surgery
    advance requests of hospital staff, 32–35
    angioplasty, 24
    bypass surgery, 15, 18, 24, 25
    preparing for, 27–32
    recovery time, 17
    stents, 24–25
    as temporary fix, 37
Sweet Potato Hash, Roasted, 257–58

talk therapy, 71–72, 132
tests, postoperative, 113–19
thallium stress test, 114
therapy, mental health, 71–72, 132
therapy, physical. *See* cardiac rehabilitation
training plan, 228–34
training plan samples
    cycling, 288–91
    swimming, 291–92
    walking, jogging, and running, 284–88
    website for updates, 283
travel
    driving, 95–98
    hotel wake-up calls, 56
    with pets, 56, 99
    by plane, 98–100
    sleep in unfamiliar environment, 56
triceps exercises, 220

triglycerides, 115–16, 155
Tuna Melt Sandwich, 262–63
turkey
    saturated fat in, 156
    Turkey Meatballs, 272–74
    Turkey Meat Loaf, 263–65
Tyras, Dennis, 188

Unbeatable stories
    acceptance of changed life (Larry Mart),
        176–77
    dying peacefully (Chase Carter),
        125–27
    following dreams (Bill Wohl), 63–65
    goal-setting (Don Monroe), 226–27
    perseverance (Yvonne Payne), 203–4
    reliance on support team (Joshua Lurie-
        Terrell), 30–32
    self-care (Mellanie True Hills), 198–99
    to share stories, 246
Unisom (doxylamine), 45
upper back exercises, 218–19
urinary catheters, 35

Vegetarian Chili, 259–60
visitors and callers
    comments by, 67, 81–83, 88–89
    control and limitation of, 29, 34, 67,
        81, 83
    overnight hospital visits, 33
visualization
    outdoor excursion, 87–88
    plane travel, 99
    resisting unhealthy foods, 167
    sex, 133
vitamin supplements, 173–78

walking
    as cardiovascular exercise, 210,
        214–16
    charity events, 227, 231, 282–83
    to digest unhealthy foods, 160
    first outdoor excursion, 85–91
    to lift depression, 71, 85
    to manage job stress, 197, 201
    to reduce anxiety, 62
    shoes for, 231
    training plan, 284–88